AGE
LESS

AGE
LESS

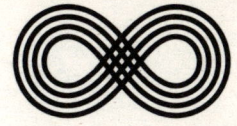

How I reduced
my biological age
from 60 to 20...
and how you can too

SANDRA PARSONS

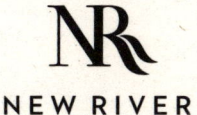

NEW RIVER

For Serge, Isabella and Luke, with love always

Disclaimer

The material in this book is for informational purposes only.
As each individual situation is unique, you should use proper
discretion, in consultation with a health care practitioner, before
undertaking the diet and techniques described in this book.
The author and publisher expressly disclaim responsibility for
any adverse effects that may result from the use or application
of the information it contains.

Published in 2025 by New River Books
Unit 105, Leroy House, 436 Essex Road, London N1 3QP
www.newriverbooks.co.uk
10 9 8 7 6 5 4 3

A CIP catalogue record for this book is available from the
British Library.
ISBN: 978-1-915780-31-7

Illustrations by Rob Brandt
Cover design by Emma Ewbank
Interior design by Smith & Gilmour

Printed and Bound in the UK using 100% Renewable Electricity
at CPI Group (UK) Ltd, Croydon, CR0 4YY.
This FSC label means that materials used for the product
have been responsibly sourced.

MIX
Paper | Supporting
responsible forestry
FSC® C013604
FSC
www.fsc.org

CONTENTS

INTRODUCTION

The quest for longevity has been going for hundreds of years, since at least the Middle Ages. Back then, alchemists believed that if they could only find the Philosopher's Stone – a mythical substance – they could use it to produce the elixir of life.

Today, not much has changed. The world's most brilliant scientists have been hired by the world's richest billionaires, from Amazon's Jeff Bezos (Altos Labs) to Google's Larry Page (California Life Company – Calico) to Paypal co-founder Peter Thiel (Methuselah Foundation), to find out if not actually how to live for ever, at least how to live healthily for a very long time indeed.

Not forgetting, of course, the redoubtable – and in my view, admirable – billionaire Bryan Johnson, who is putting vast amounts of his money into cutting-edge longevity research using his own body (and with astonishing results so far).

Meanwhile, longevity clinics are opening in the world's richest capital cities. London alone boasts several at the time of writing, from the Hooke in Mayfair, where the top-tier membership is currently £54,000 per year – entirely affordable by the financiers who live and work there – to the (slightly) more accessible Solice around the corner, where annual membership comes in at just under £10,000.

The average age of Hooke's clientele is 49. A top-tier membership gives you twice-yearly medical, cognitive, nutritional, fitness and wellbeing reviews as well as a host of other appraisals, including blood tests, sleep assessments and your biological age score, plus personalised supplements.

For those wanting maximum access to longevity expertise while on holiday, there are premium retreats in some of the world's most luxurious destinations. In 2024, Kate Moss was among the gilded few who flew to Thailand for a five-day retreat at RAKxa with Deepak Chopra – 'For optimal wellness… where ancient wisdom combines with cutting edge medicine'.

For £17,000, guests enjoyed six treatments a day in addition to longevity talks from Chopra.(I should say here that I am a huge fan of Deepak Chopra. Asked by someone at that same retreat to give his tips for a better life, he replied: 'There's only one. Take it easy… disengage from the drama.' You could argue there's invaluable wisdom in that reply, because letting go is one of the most important longevity practices there is. If you can do that, you will massively reduce your anxiety and stress – one of the greatest obstacles to living a long and healthy life.)

Nevertheless, you would be forgiven for thinking that when it comes to longevity it's a rich man's (or woman's) world.

Well, I have cheering news. It doesn't matter if you can't afford any of the above. Because the great thing about scientists is that most of them publish their research, and make it available, if not for free then for not much more than US$30 per paper.

And I am here to tell you that *all* of us can adopt their methods and their advice for very little money. Sure, it is great to do the tests. But you can achieve the same results for an awful lot less.

The alchemists of the Middle Ages speculated that if they ever did manage to identify that elusive Philosopher's Stone, it would be a common substance, found everywhere but unappreciated.

Seven centuries on, it turns out that in that respect at least they may have been right. Because, while the elixir of youth has yet to materialise, what science is discovering in the meantime is that the human body has an almost infinite capacity to heal itself.

The secret to living a longer, healthier life is actually within each and every one of us. All we have to do is allow the body to do its work. And that's where this book comes in.

Try following my Age Less reset plan for just three weeks, and watch a miracle begin.

* * *

Imagine being 100 and feeling like a lithe, energetic 60-year-old. Or turning 80 and being in the same shape as a fit 50-year-old.

Some of the world's most brilliant and respected longevity scientists believe this is entirely achievable – not in some utopian future, but right now.

I happen to believe the scientists are right.

What's more, achieving it doesn't involve weird injections or expensive equipment, merely changing some simple habits.

How do I know this? Because after several years of changing my own habits, I took one of the most accurate tests available to find out my biological age.

My actual chronological age was 60. My biological age was 20.

That's right. I was 60 on the outside and 20 on the inside.

The secret of how I got to be four decades younger isn't really a secret at all. It's just the result of having read dozens of books and papers from the world's leading longevity scientists over the years and adopting the best of their suggestions.

I passionately believe that it is possible to age not just gracefully but with increased vitality and zest for life. Entering my 60s I feel more alive than I ever have, fizzing with enthusiasm and energy.

According to David Sinclair, professor of genetics at Harvard Medical School and one of the world's leading experts on ageing, only 20 per cent of our longevity is down to our genes. The rest – a whopping 80 per cent – is down to our environment and our behaviour.

In other words, your future health is largely in your own hands.

As we age, most of us eventually come to a fork in the road. Something happens – an injury, a chronic disease or perhaps just a slow slippage into general frailty and fatigue – and we have to make a choice. We can either slide into gradual decline and ill health, in the fatalistic but misguided belief that this is the inevitable consequence of getting older. Or we can decide to take charge of our life, our health and our future and do something about it.

MY STORY

Until the age of 43 I smoked and did no exercise. I wasn't overweight but my diet was poor – lots of ready meals, a chocolate bar a day. I drank a glass or two of wine most nights to unwind.

A mother of two young children, I also worked full-time in a very stressful job that involved lots of pressure. I slept badly, had crippling migraines and shoulders like rocks.

In short, I felt rubbish. And I remained in this state for a very long time – years. Not surprisingly, I was permanently exhausted.

If you'd said to me then that just by changing how I ate, moved and rested I could maintain the same workload while feeling incredible, I would have laughed in disbelief and said you were crazy.

I had absolutely no time or desire to think about changing any of those things – it was taking all my energy just to keep going.

If that's how you feel now, take heart. Believe me, you can make those changes and you will feel so much better. You just have to have faith, and take it one step at a time.

Looking back, in my case it all began with an injury – one that could so easily have ended with my becoming immobile and even more unhealthy than I already was.

My sister-in-law had been talking about running, which she loved, and said it might be a good stress reliever for me. I told her I didn't think I could run even to the end of the road. She suggested I try a short jog to the church and back, just to see. The total distance couldn't have been more than half a mile. It turned out that even that was too much for me. I was gasping for breath after just a minute or two and had to stop. But I have a stubborn streak and tend to be competitive with myself, so I carried on for a few weeks, three mornings a week at 6.30am, until one morning I managed to get there and back again without collapsing.

And that's when it happened. A deep, deep pain in my lower back. By the time I drove the children to school 90 minutes later I was in agony. On the Tube to work I realised very quickly that this was not going to wear off; not only could I not sit down because of the pain, but I couldn't stand, either. It was a 45-minute journey which I endured by alternating between standing and sitting. The pain was so intense that occasionally – to the bemusement of other passengers who stared but, this being London public transport, said not a word – I couldn't help groaning out loud.

By around 4pm, the pain had spread all over my back and down the whole of my right leg. A kind colleague drove me to her osteopath, who told me my entire back had gone into spasm to protect itself from whatever it was that had happened. The pain was extreme, far exceeding anything I'd experienced in childbirth (and I say that as someone who gave birth the second time with no pain relief at all).

I have had many reasons over the years to be beyond thankful I am married to a doctor. I phoned him to tell him what was happening and that evening he came home with some extremely strong medication. For the first time in 14 hours, the agony faded away. It felt like a miracle.

But when I didn't take the medication, the pain remained excruciating. My leg stayed numb for a week; I struggled to walk at anything faster than a snail's pace. An MRI scan showed a curvature, or scoliosis, on my spine that unbeknownst to me had been there since birth (meaning that without good core strength my back was simply an accident waiting to happen) and a severe prolapsed disc.

Several doctors advised an operation. I didn't like the idea and my husband's view was to avoid surgery if possible. So I began my long, slow recovery by following the advice of Sara Key[1] – a brilliant osteopath who also happens to have helped both King Charles and Queen Camilla – to rock gently on my back with my knees hugged into my chest, and then to progress to gently extending it by lying on a yoga block.

As the weeks turned into months, I gradually regained more and more function, although the outside edge of my right foot remained stubbornly numb and it was six or seven years before I recovered full movement in all my toes.

---

1 If you have back trouble I highly recommend her excellent book, *Sarah Key's Back Sufferers' Bible*

About six months after that agonising injury, I started Pilates, to strengthen my core. I found I enjoyed it. And a few months after that I finally gave up smoking.

I should say here that I didn't give up smoking in order to feel better. In fact, I LOVED smoking. I smoked for almost 30 years! It was the one thing that gave me a tiny bit of 'me time' – a little treat, just a few minutes to myself.

But the British government was about to introduce a new law making it illegal to smoke indoors. I didn't want to sit in a café or bar knowing I couldn't have a longed-for cigarette with my coffee or glass of wine. And for years I'd felt guilty about the terrible example I was setting my children, who at the time were five and 10.

Then, through my job, the opportunity came up to meet Paul McKenna, who offered to help me stop. You can call it fate, or the universe sending help, or simple serendipity.

Either way, even though I found the idea of giving up terrifying, and in any case didn't believe I could properly stop (I'd quit each time I was pregnant – easily, thanks to acute morning sickness – but each time started again several months after the birth), I decided to try. And no one was more surprised than me to discover when I left the session with Paul McKenna that I simply didn't want a cigarette. I'd imagined I would want one straight away, or at least with my next coffee. Instead, I felt amazing – joyously alive – with no desire to smoke at all.

Although I didn't realise it at the time, I was now firmly on the path of transformation.

I continued with Pilates, and eventually gained enough confidence to start running again. I also took up yoga. After just a few years, I found I was exercising almost every day and feeling astonishingly good on it. From there it was just a short step to time-restricted eating and a myriad other changes, including becoming fanatical about sleep and learning how to give myself deep rest and relaxation whenever I need it.

We are all different, so for you that first step on the path to transformation could be something else. It could be weaning yourself off your morning croissant, or getting off the train or bus a stop or two early to walk, or learning to play padel or eating more vegetables every day or starting yoga… it doesn't really matter what it is, to be honest. What matters is that you start the process of change, in whatever way you can manage.

Had I not decided to start taking responsibility for my own health by doing everything I could to heal my back injury, I could easily have ended up with permanent crippling pain. I might well have become dependent on medication. I wouldn't have felt able to walk much, let alone started to experience the fantastic benefits that regular exercise brings. I could have given up, but instead I decided to bite the bullet. Or, to use another expression that I find helpful, I chose my hard.

And I encourage you to choose your hard too. Yes, it's hard to make a change – whether that's to quit smoking or to stop eating crisps and biscuits or to start going to the gym.

But the alternative is also hard. In fact, it's harder.

It's hard to be unfit. It's hard to be overweight. It's hard to have crippling migraines. It's hard to have shoulders that ache. It's hard to wake up every morning feeling you can barely lift your head off the pillow, let alone summon the energy to climb out of bed.

It's hard feeling tired all the time.

So – choose your hard. Because you'll find that choosing the hard that makes you fitter, leaner, stronger, younger is the hard that, over time, becomes the easy.

OK, maybe not easy. But easier. A lot, lot easier.

And that's how it came about that a few years ago, still working long hours in a full-time stressful office job, and with an elderly widowed father to look after to boot, I opened the email with the result of the test for my biological age.

Good news, Sandra, it read. Your biological age is 20.

Just to remind you, my actual – chronological – age was 60.

And if I can do it, you can too. I'm going to show you how.

THE RESET PLAN

As I said before, a longer, healthier life comes down to changing simple habits that will keep you younger.

None of the three changes I list below require complicated calculations or planning. The very opposite. Rather, they are about doing what comes naturally to us – returning to behaviours that humans have evolved over thousands of years.

1. **Eat 10 per cent less.** That's right, just 10 per cent. It doesn't sound like much – because it isn't. It's the equivalent of a small portion of McDonald's fries, or three small chocolate chip cookies. Believe it or not, science now shows that's all it takes to set in train incredible health and longevity gains, from improving your cardiovascular health to decreasing your risk of type 2 diabetes and dementia, while also reducing your biological age and losing weight. I will show you two easy but powerfully effective ways of doing this.

2. **Move more.** This idea may make you groan, but it is crucial for your mental and cognitive health as well as your physical

fitness. Exercise is as vital for your brain as it is for your heart. Plus it makes you feel GREAT. Honestly. Please try my plan and see for yourself. You don't have to be remotely fit or sporty to start (as I've already explained, I certainly wasn't) and anyone can do it.

3. **Rest more deeply.** This is mainly about achieving quality sleep, but it's also about being able to get deep rest during the day when you need it. You may think you can't. You may protest that you don't have time, or that you've tried everything and nothing works. Trust me – you can rest more, and longer. You will not only sleep better, you will find it easier to get back to sleep too. And I will also show you an amazing and incredibly easy way to completely re-energise during the day whenever you need to, in as little as 15 minutes.

These three changes revolutionised my life, and they will revolutionise yours.

My simple, three-step plan takes just three weeks to complete. And it is easy to follow and can be done by anyone. It doesn't matter how overweight you are, how unfit, how sleepless, how old. It is never too late – although, as with all new health regimes, I suggest that before you begin you check first with your doctor if you have any concerns.

Why three weeks? Because that's all it takes to feel a hugely transformational effect – and that's what will give you the incentive and the momentum to keep going. Three weeks is enough time to reset your body so that it starts to adapt to new ways of eating, moving and resting. It will then be much easier for you to continue on the path to a longer, healthier life. Your body will start to lose old cravings and begin to recognise that this new way feels better.

The changes may only be small at first, but they will be tangible. You will find that you want fewer sugary snacks. You will notice how good it feels to move more. And you will wake up feeling more rested.

And my bet is that, after completing the plan, you will feel so well and full of energy that you will want to continue. You may not stick to it utterly consistently, but you will have sown a seed of change that you will want to nurture.

Remember, the results are cumulative: a bit like compound interest on savings, if you consistently make small lifestyle adjustments day after day, you will see improvements every week and month, amounting to a huge change after a year. You will have more vitality, you will move with more ease and flexibility, feel and look better – firmer, leaner, stronger. And afterwards, even if you decide to follow the plan for just one week every month, you will still see extraordinary changes and improvements to your health and wellbeing.

Of course, there will be days when, despite your best intentions, things go wrong. Maybe you skip a workout, or you eat rubbish food, or have a really bad night's sleep. Maybe all three. Don't worry. It doesn't mean you've failed. It's what happens from time to time: a blip. And it's not just you, either: we all have them.

What matters is not the blip, but how you choose to react to it. You can decide that the blip is proof that this was all a terrible idea, that you don't want to live longer and be healthier anyway. Or you can tell yourself that it's just a temporary setback, nothing to panic about – and get right back to the plan wherever you left off.

Just keep going. In a few weeks you will not only start to see and feel improvements in yourself, but most importantly of all, you will have more confidence and self-belief. You can do this – one step at a time.

HOW TO USE THIS BOOK

First, I will introduce you to the world's leading longevity scientists, whose groundbreaking research, dogged hard work and brilliant thinking has informed and underpinned every change I have made.

Then we will get straight on with the plan. Each step starts with a brief questionnaire, designed to help you see where you are now. Being clear about exactly what you're eating, how you're moving and what kind of sleep you are currently having is important if you are to change and get better. There are no right or wrong answers – but the more honest you are with yourself, the easier it will be for you to chart your progress and see some real improvements in every aspect of your life, not just physically but mentally and emotionally too.

Once you've identified your current patterns of eating, moving and sleeping, you will be ready to start. There is a three-week reset plan for each step. You can do all the plans together, taking three weeks to change your eating, moving and sleeping all at the same time. Or you can start with just one step – for example, food – and do that reset plan, before moving on to the next. It's completely up to you – just choose what feels right for you.

Scattered throughout the reset plan are 'lifelines' – quick hits designed to give you a boost when you're struggling and need an easy win. Towards the end of the book, there are some short but useful chapters on how to combat stress, how to make a habit stick, and tweaks you can make to optimise your health according to your particular needs, whether that's with vitamins, minerals or other supplements, including hormones (such as HRT). Of course, you can also choose to do without any of those things.

I
WHY WE AGE

Warning to those who hated science at school: some science-y bits coming up. Feel free to skip this chapter, if that sort of stuff bores you. The short version is: our lifestyle makes us age. It is the underlying cause of many of the diseases we associate with 'old age': type 2 diabetes, stroke, heart attack, dementia, to name just four. Our bodies are perfectly capable of keeping us healthier for much longer. But poor diet, lack of exercise and insufficient sleep and rest switch off or impair many of our inbuilt repair mechanisms. Change our lifestyle and we can slow down ageing, hugely reduce our chances of those diseases and live longer, healthier, fuller lives.

THE 'INFORMATION THEORY OF AGEING'

To understand why we age, we need first to have a short lesson in epigenetics.

We each have about 20,000 genes – these being segments of our DNA, the strings of molecules needed for our cells to function. And the information within our genes needs to be read in order for our cells to be able to use it properly. This 'reading' of gene information is the function of the epigenome. And it is changes within the epigenome that, according to a new theory conceived by David Sinclair, the Australian-American biologist and professor of genetics I mentioned in the introduction, are the real reason we age.

Basically, as we go through life, some of our genes begin to change their structure because of epigenetic disruption – change or damage at a cellular level, caused by things like a poor diet, excessive stress or environmental pollution.

Epigenetic changes, just to be clear, are down to us. They are changes that happen not because our DNA itself has changed, but because outside factors in our environment – such as how we eat, sleep and move – have disrupted the way our genes work. Effectively, the gene information that our cells receive and depend on becomes confused. Professor Sinclair calls it the 'Information Theory of Ageing'.

As I stated before, how long we live is determined only partly by our genes – they are responsible for as little as one-fifth of our longevity. The rest is up to us: the way we live determines how well our genes function, which in turn determines how well our cells perform.

Imagine for a moment that your body is a car. Now imagine that the electrical system of the car has started to go wrong and that the windscreen wipers come on even when it's not raining. A fault has occurred, and you can't turn them off. So they are constantly going back and forth across a dry windscreen.

Eventually, the rubber starts to erode, so that when it does actually rain, the wipers are no longer effective at wiping the water away, which means you can no longer drive the car safely.

Epigenetic changes effect similar disruptions in your body. The wrong genes come on at the wrong time and in the wrong place. Cells begin to age and die. This is what causes ageing on every level: weaker muscles, wrinkly skin, arthritis, dementia and chronic diseases from heart failure to cancer. And on it goes – until eventually we die.

And then there is inflammation, which plays another key role.

WHY INFLAMMATION MATTERS

When we have an acute infection, or injury, our body reacts fast. It sends cortisol to the area, and increases production of white blood cells in an attempt to fight off the infection.

This response is crucial for our health and survival and results in 'good' inflammation. For example, when we cut ourselves or have a bad bump, the injured area becomes red and sore – inflamed. It means the white blood cells and cortisol are fighting to prevent infection or injury spreading.

Then, once the repairs are underway, the inflammation gradually lessens and eventually disappears.

But when acute injuries or infections pile up repeatedly, the inflammation doesn't disappear. Instead, it can become chronic, constantly 'on', weakening our immune system and reducing our ability to fight disease.

Most chronic diseases are underpinned by inflammation, from heart disease to type 2 diabetes to dementia, Alzheimer's and some cancers.

This chronic inflammation can have many other causes too. Sleep deprivation and chronic stress are both factors, as is eating a diet high in processed foods and sugar and low in vegetables.

So far, so scary. However... as many leading longevity scientists are now demonstrating, ageing is not inevitable. It is simply a disease – one that science is discovering is treatable. More than that, it can be reversed. And one of the best ways to do that is by putting ourselves under stress – the right kind of stress, that is.

A surprising way to reduce inflammation (and reduce your chances of a heart attack or stroke)

If you want to live longer, it's crucial that you brush your teeth regularly – and floss them too. Many studies show the link between poor oral health and the risk of heart disease, with chronic inflammation thought to be the cause. One study, by researchers at University College London in 2010,[1] which defined good oral hygiene as brushing teeth twice a day, found that those who brushed once a day had a 30 per cent increased risk of cardiovascular disease, while those who brushed rarely had a 70 per cent increased risk. And a preliminary study presented by the American Heart Association at its annual conference in February 2025 found that teeth flossing was associated with a 22 per cent lower risk of ischemic stroke, 44 per cent lower risk of cardioembolic stroke (blood clots travelling from the heart) and 12 per cent lower risk of arterial fibrillation. To the researchers' surprise, this lower risk was independent of regular brushing and routine dental visits or other oral hygiene behaviours.[2]

1 Toothbrushing, inflammation, and risk of cardiovascular disease, *BMJ*, 2010 – www.bmj.com/content/340/bmj.c2451
2 Regular dental flossing may lower risk of stroke from blood clots, irregular heartbeats, *ScienceDaily*, 2025 – www.sciencedaily.com/releases/2025/01/250130161704.htm

THE RIGHT KIND OF STRESS

The most important principle to accept when it comes to optimising your health – and with it, your longevity – is to be prepared to feel uncomfortable. Basically, you need to trick your body and brain into thinking they need to work harder to survive.

The scientific word for this adversity process is hormesis. When we put our bodies into adversity, our cells go into survival mode, conserving energy where possible, killing off cells that aren't essential and shutting down reproduction. And then, when the stress ends, the cells crank into high gear, renewing, repairing, reproducing and rebooting our entire system in the process.

As humans, we are built to withstand stress to survive. The problem is that today we have none of those drivers that we were conditioned for thousands of years to accept.

Back in our hunter-gatherer days, we had to take food where we could find it. We needed to conserve our supplies, and our strength. We had to hunt. We had to walk or run long distances to find, kill or gather food, and to defend our supplies. We had to accept that sometimes, according to the weather or the time of year, there wouldn't be enough to eat.

However, modern life in the Western world is designed to give us as much convenience and comfort as possible. Indeed, in the last hundred years or so, we have had such easy access to abundant food and security that we have distorted our evolutionary function. Within minutes of feeling hungry we can find food, ready-made and ready to eat. We don't have to move much. We don't have to fight for it.

Because this constant abundance is such a recent development in our history, our bodies have not evolved to deal with it. We are still conditioned to grab food whenever we can, the tastier and more calorie-rich the better.

So it's no wonder we find ourselves automatically reaching for that burger or almond croissant – that's the result of thousands of years of evolution, designed to help us survive. Except that now it is doing precisely the opposite.

Today there is so much fat-laden, sugary food, so easily available, that we have become obese and unfit, stuffing our bodies full of convenience foods and chemicals. We are killing ourselves.

If we are serious about living longer, we need to force our body, every day, into some sort of DIScomfort. This is what hormesis is all about. And the two most important ways to do this are to eat a little less and move a little more.

When we fast, for example, we start sending signals to our brain that perhaps food is not so abundant. The body prepares for possible scarcity by shutting down whichever parts of its system it temporarily doesn't need, running on the least energy possible. It is tricked into thinking it has to go into starvation mode, and cells then start eating themselves to survive, as no energy is coming into the body from the outside. But the cells only eat the parts of themselves that no longer function well, leaving the functioning parts available to be recycled and reused once food enters the system again. The scientific word for this is autophagy. It comes from Greek: *autos* (self) and *phagomai* (to eat) – literally, self eating.

Then, when we eat again, the body goes into overdrive, replacing, repairing and renewing cells, which in turn means we become healthier, stronger, and yes – younger.

The same is true of exercise. If we are barely moving, we take in more calories than we need and also allow our muscles to fall into disuse. But once we start using them, say by lots of brisk walking, running, cycling or lifting heavy weights, we begin to stress our muscle fibres, as well as our hearts and lungs. Then, when they are allowed to rest, they too begin the process of repairing and renewing, ready for the next onslaught.

If your reaction to both these ideas is fear – relax. That's a perfectly normal response – after all, these things are only of benefit *because* they stress your body.

It's even true for temperature. It is wonderfully beneficial to your body (and brain) to expose yourself to extreme cold (just a few minutes a day, three days a week) and extreme heat. Three or four minutes' cold water swimming, for example, produces a huge surge of dopamine, the feelgood neurotransmitter. You will feel extraordinarily energised and positive for at least two or three hours. It's better than any drug – and it's free.

The point is, what doesn't kill you really does make you stronger.

The more you do things that stress your body, the better you will feel – and the better your brain will feel. You will be surprised how quickly you stop fearing – and maybe even enjoy – eating less and moving more.

And here's the beautiful thing. The reset plan not only gives you some of that right kind of stress. It will also dissolve the constant low-lying stress you suffer from having too much work, too many late nights, relationship angst – piece by piece, day by day, until one morning you wake up and realise that the nagging headache, the bloated stomach, the rock-solid shoulders and the nameless fear lurking somewhere in your subconscious… have simply melted away.

You will find it easier to eat a little more healthily. As you start to exercise more, you will begin to sleep better. As you sleep better you will feel more energised and less inclined to reach for the instant hit of fast, ultra-processed food. Before you know it, your life will be so much simpler and easier – and you will be healthier and more relaxed. Chronic inflammation will subside. Your epigenome will be less disrupted. And you will be on the path to achieving what this book is all about – not just living longer, but living longer as healthily as possible – strong, resilient and flexible in body and in mind.

WHY AGEING IS NOT INEVITABLE

According to the American longevity expert Dr Mark Hyman, one of the main reasons a three-year-old can run around with boundless energy for hours while a 90-year-old moves very slowly is due to the number of healthy mitochondria they have (mitochondria are the energy factories that power our cells).

This is not a new idea. More than 50 years ago, when Dr Hyman and indeed many of the world's top longevity scientists were still children (and some not even born), an American scientist called Denham Harman published a groundbreaking paper, in which he proposed that the reason we age is that over time, our mitochondria become severely damaged by free radicals.

Free radicals are atoms or molecules that have become unstable or out of control. Molecules are made up of two or more bonded atoms, and are the building blocks of every single thing on earth. Atoms, meanwhile, are made up of protons, neutrons and electrons. For an atom to be stable, its electrons, which are like mini forcefields of energy, need to be paired. However, sometimes this bond will weaken and an electron will 'go rogue', leaving its molecule and attaching to another one, thereby creating two unstable molecules or free radicals. As each stable molecule is attacked by one of these rogue electrons, it becomes unstable itself, setting off a chain reaction that leads to cell damage and destruction. This is one cause of ageing; and each cell in our body is bombarded with thousands of hits from free radicals every day.

Some free radicals are generated as part of normal cell function, such as detoxification, while others are produced by mistake, or in reaction to environmental factors such as pollution or sunburn or cigarette smoke.

The good news is that the body has a remedy for this, in the form of antioxidants. Antioxidants work by freeing electrons and pairing them again, making the atoms and molecules stable once more. Powerful antioxidants are found in many of the plant foods we eat – broccoli, spinach, carrots and strawberries, to name just a few.

So the more antioxidants we consume the better. (For more information on how to increase your antioxidants, see p74).

Since Denham Harman's paper in 1972, the field of longevity science has come a long way. And many of its leading experts, including Dr Mark Hyman, Dr David Sinclair and Dr Valter Longo, professor of gerontology and biological sciences and director of the University of Southern California Longevity Institute in LA, believe that ageing is a disease – or at least, that it can be treated like a disease. And one that we can partially reverse.

Our bodies are designed both to clean up and repair old cells and proteins and also to build new molecules, cells and tissues. 'The problem with ageing is imbalance: too much decay and not enough rebuilding,' says Dr Hyman. 'If we do not take care of ourselves, if we do not activate our healing programmes and longevity switches, if we go about our business as usual, the diseases of ageing will take hold and degrade our bodies over time.'

The main lifestyle behaviours that affect the body's ability to heal and rebuild are eating too much of the wrong kind of food; lack of exercise; and too little sleep and restorative rest.

David Sinclair points out that research into almost every living organism, from yeast to fruit flies, to mice and rhesus monkeys, has proved that reducing your caloric intake by 30 per cent increases your lifespan. In the case of rhesus monkeys, it has been shown to prolong life to the human equivalent of 120 years.

Dr Longo has studied caloric restriction for more than three decades, and has done more research into humans and fasting than perhaps any other scientist today. He is clear that, with the right nutrition and fasting, we can optimise our chances of staying fully functional into our 90s, 100s and beyond.

'One of the primary ways to achieve this is to exploit our body's innate ability to regenerate itself at the cellular and organ levels,' he says.

Although our continual consumption and unhealthy modern diet in the Western world has kept our body's regeneration mechanisms switched off, he has discovered they can be switched back on again – quite easily.

He explains that research – not just his own but many other studies too – shows that the body only goes into full-blown autophagy (which he likens to pulling down the damaged part of an old building and rebuilding it from scratch with new materials) after five days of fasting. Of course, doing such an extreme form of fasting is difficult and potentially dangerous. So, instead, he has developed the Fasting Mimicking Diet (FMD), which tricks the body into thinking it's fasting, while at the same time giving it all the macro- and micronutrients it needs. Randomised, clinically controlled trials have shown this has astonishing effects on health, reversing diabetes, improving recovery from cancer, cardiovascular diseases and autoimmune disorders and even – in a pilot study of 13 people with chronic kidney disease published in October 2024 – improved kidney function, possibly by activating the same regenerative process they have demonstrated for rats in which kidneys are severely damaged.[1]

In an ideal world, according to Dr Longo, people would do three cycles of his FMD diet a year. (A study[2] in 2024 showed that three cycles of FMD reduce biological age by 2.5 years.)

It's worth noting that the FMD, which is posted to you with three pre-packaged meals for each of the five days, plus snacks, is expensive – £179 at the time of writing. However, Dr Longo takes no salary or fee from L-Nutra, the company that makes it, and has been donating 100 per cent of his salary and the income from shares to the Create Cures Foundation in LA, a non-profit longevity and nutritional centre founded by him in 2015.

According to Longo, the best way to force our bodies into a slower ageing plus repair and regenerative mode is by having a low (but sufficient) protein, normal-calorie, mostly-pescatarian 'longevity diet', with periodic cycles of the fasting mimicking diet.

He himself hopes to live to 120. (To put this into context, as of September 2023, life expectancy in the UK from birth was 83.6 years for females and 79.9 years for males.) When I meet him at the Longevity Institute at the University of Southern California, he is a lean and energetic 56, and takes the several flights of stairs up to his office at pace.

'Of course, any of us could die tomorrow for whatever reason,' he says easily. 'For example, you could end up with a neuroblastoma

---

1 A kidney-specific fasting-mimicking diet induces podocyte reprogramming and restores renal function in glomerulopathy, *Science Translational Med.*, 2024 – www.science.org/doi/10.1126/scitranslmed.adl5514
2 Fasting-mimicking diet causes hepatic and blood markers changes indicating reduced biological age and disease risk. *Nature Comms.*, 2024. www.nature.com/articles/s41467-024-45260-9

that's got nothing to do with your diet or exercise and that's it, that's your fate and you're going to die. But I think it's good to have this 120-year plan and say "Look, I'll do everything that's going to get me there."

'We think of poor nutrition, lack of exercise and the genes we inherit from our parents as the major risk factors for diseases. But by monitoring the age at which people are diagnosed with different diseases, we know that *ageing itself* is the main risk factor for cancer, cardiovascular disease, Alzheimer's and many other diseases.

'The probability that a 20-year-old woman will develop breast cancer within the next 10 years of her life is roughly 1 in 2000. The risk is 1 in 24 for a 70-year-old woman – that's an increase by almost a factor of 100.

'If ageing is the central risk factor for all major diseases, it's much smarter to intervene on ageing itself than to try to prevent and treat diseases one by one. Few people know, for example, that curing cancer or cardiac disease today would increase the average lifespan by only a little over three years.'

Let's just think about that for a moment. You are almost 100 times more likely to develop breast cancer when you are 70 than when you are 20. Why? Because of ageing.

But here's the great thing: it's never too late! As a remarkable 2023 study[3] of data from nearly half a million British participants showed, if you switch from an unhealthy diet to an optimally healthy one (rich in beans, wholegrains, vegetables, nuts and fruit and low in red meat and sugary drinks) aged 40, you can gain another *10 years* of life expectancy; and even if you wait until you're

---

3 Life expectancy can increase by up to 10 years following sustained shifts towards healthier diets in the United Kingdom. *Nature Food*, 2023
www.nature.com/articles/s43016-023-00868-w

70 before making that change, you can gain another *five years*.

So I hope you need no more persuading that one of the best ways to force our bodies into repair mode, or hormesis, is by restricting our calories. And as I've already mentioned, I am going to provide you with an incredibly easy way of achieving this.

But we also need to be getting more exercise, rest and sleep – and doing what we can to lessen stress.

Exercise increases our mitochondria, improves our overall heart health (turn to p97 to find out how one exercise regime rejuvenated the hearts of middle-aged people), decreases 'bad' cholesterol, enhances sugar control, and speeds up the process of autophagy. Stressing our body with exercise encourages cells to renew and repair in the same way that fasting does.

Meanwhile, lack of sleep increases our risk of dementia, cancer, heart disease, stroke and diabetes. Regularly sleeping less than six hours a night means you are three times more likely to have hardened arteries, as well as being more prone to Alzheimer's and dementia. And if you're over 45, it also means you have three times the risk of a heart attack or strokes.

According to Matthew Walker, a professor of neuroscience at Berkeley who has studied sleep for more than 20 years (and wrote a superb book about it – *Why We Sleep*), there have been more than 20 large-scale studies, tracking millions of people over many years, which all report the same thing: the shorter someone sleeps, the shorter their life.

A third of us regularly get less than the recommended seven hours. In addition, lack of sleep is likely to make us stressed – another cause of early death. One study in Finland found that heavy stress (defined as stress perceived as being greater than that of most people) shortened men's lives by almost three years. And prolonged stress increases the risk of heart disease, addiction and mood disorders. Just as being well rested means we feel more able to tackle daily life, so too does reducing stress. A study at Yale University using an epigenetic clock to measure participants' biological age found that those who reported the most stress had accelerated ageing markers.

Eating well, sleeping well and exercising regularly will all help reduce stress. But nothing is as effective in my experience as sitting perfectly still for 10–20 minutes, with your eyes closed. Many people are daunted by the idea of 'meditation' – you don't have to call it that; you can just think of it as sitting in stillness.

The idea is to let go of tension – much of which we cause ourselves, by overthinking. You can't stop thinking, but with practice you can stop getting so involved with your thoughts. Many people find it helpful to count each inhale and exhale, up to 10, and then repeat.

The purpose of sitting like this is to quieten the mind and connect with the inner 'you' or self – the one that has nothing to

Just one cigarette?

It goes without saying that smoking is one of the quickest ways to shorten your life. But if you're someone who protests you're only a social smoker, or prides yourself on smoking just one a day, it might be worth paying attention to this statement from Professor Bill Kraus, a cardiologist at Duke University in North Carolina: 'I have worked with the Environmental Protection Agency in the US on the role of air pollution on all kinds of cardiovascular risk. One factoid I hold with me and share with my patients... one cigarette a day, ONE, carries the same level of cardiopulmonary risk as exposure to the **worst** air pollution **daily**.'

do with your sex, age, job or lifestyle. Those who experience its profound effects return to it again and again. And many studies have shown its beneficial effects on depression and anxiety.

WILL WE ONE DAY BE ABLE TO REVERSE AGEING?

In his 2019 book *Lifespan*, David Sinclair revealed he is working on a form of cellular reprogramming that he believes will result in us being able to reverse ageing with one injection.

It would involve getting a jab at the age of 30 with a specially engineered adeno-associated virus, or AAV, which would carry a small number of genes that could be turned on with something like a common antibiotic.

Nothing would happen until your mid-40s, which is when you normally feel the first effects of ageing. Then a course of the antibiotic would be prescribed, which would switch on the reprogramming genes.

'Over the next month,' writes Dr Sinclair, 'your body would undergo a rejuvenation process. Grey hair would disappear. Wounds would heal faster, wrinkles would fade. Organs would regenerate. You would think faster, hear higher-pitched sounds, and no longer need glasses to read a menu. Your body would feel young again.'

Then, when the antibiotic course ended, the reprogramming would stop. You would continue your life for the next few decades – and then have another course to rejuvenate you again.

Dr Sinclair is aware this sounds like science fiction. His response? 'Let me be clear: it is not.'

Since his laboratory has already been celebrated for achieving what was previously thought impossible – regenerating the optic nerve in mice, restoring vision and potentially ending age-related macular degeneration and glaucoma in humans – I take what he says very seriously indeed.

The test I took

Many DNA age tests analyse how gene expression is influenced by lifestyle and environment to determine biological age.

Unlike those tests, GlycanAge specifically focuses on measuring chronic inflammation in the body.

While acute inflammation can be beneficial – the body's short-term response to repair damage caused by a particular stressor – chronic inflammation is extremely harmful. Constant activation means white blood cells are continually deployed, even when there's no real threat. This confuses the immune response, making it either overactive or sluggish, both of which are problematic.

As I've already explained, this chronic inflammation plays an important role in many age-related diseases, from heart disease, stroke, cancer, dementia, diabetes and renal failure to autoimmune conditions like rheumatoid arthritis and lupus.

The GlycanAge test measures glycans, which are powerful biomarkers of chronic inflammation/ageing. Each of us has literally billions of them – they are in every cell in our bodies.

Based on the type of glycans that can be found on our immunoglobulin G (IgG), the most abundant protein in our immune system, says Dr Julija Juric of GlycanAge, we can get a fairly clear picture of how well someone is ageing. Large epidemiological studies have revealed that glycans change more than ten years before diseases like heart failure, stroke or diabetes actually manifest.

Not only this, but glycans have also been found to regulate chronic inflammation, meaning that you can actually change your biological age by changing your lifestye. 'With a simple change in diet, exercise routine and sleep pattern, you can significantly impact your biological age,' says Dr Juric.

In the meantime, his research shows that certain supplements, in particular nicotinamide mononucleotide, or NMN for short, can have even more beneficial effects than fasting. This is controversial and at the time of writing there are only a few small studies in humans showing some benefit (although there are plenty on mice). For more on this, turn to Chapter 6.

THE THREE-STEP RESET

My three-step reset plan addresses the three key elements that are the foundation stones of longevity: eating less, moving more, resting better. There is a three-week plan for each step, involving gentle, progressive change, with added extra options for those who might be further down the longevity path than others or want more of a challenge.

As I said earlier, you can either go 'all in' and do all three plans at once, or you can do them more methodically and slowly, one by one.

It's up to you, and it partly comes down to what sort of personality you have. But as long as you complete each three-week plan, whether concurrently or consecutively, you will reap the benefits.

Just to recap: eating less and moving more stresses the body in ways that cause it to create new cells and replenish or ditch old ones, making you stronger, leaner and more energetic.

The third step, deep rest, is also vital for your health and longevity. However, it works slightly differently from the other two, in that it does not involve the process of hormesis, where you put your body and brain into adversity in order to trick them into thinking they need to work harder in order to survive.

That kind of stress is good for us. However, nature needs balance, and so we also have to allow them to recover, as it is only then that the repair and rejuvenation processes can begin. The most effective way to do that is through sleep; though there are other ways you can get deep rest in short bursts during the day which are hugely healing for the brain and body – I will describe them in Chapter 4.

The world's leading longevity experts all agree on the three basic principles of eating less, moving more and resting better. But navigating a path through all the research and getting to grips with the science is a complicated task. The terms can be confusing and the material very dense. This is where I can help.

I've spent years following the developments in what is one of the most dynamic and fastest-growing areas of science today, and applied them to make huge improvements to my own health and longevity. Now I want to share what I've learned with you, so that you can do the same.

So, let's get started! The path to living longer and more healthily, with more energy and more joy, begins right here. You are just 21 days and three steps away from becoming younger, stronger, leaner and fitter.

2

EATING LESS

The most consistent point on which longevity experts agree is that caloric restriction – eating less – prolongs life in humans.

But, as we discovered in Chapter 1, most studies on the subject (and there are many, dating all the way back to the 1930s) have been done on the basis of a 30 per cent reduction. In other words, eating almost a third less. And for most people that's a totally unrealistic and unsustainable goal, no matter how many extra years of life they might gain.

So I have good news. The most comprehensive and extensive study ever done on caloric restriction in humans shows that actually you only have to cut your calories by 10–12 per cent to drastically reduce your biological age, and improve everything from your cardiovascular health to your risk of diabetes and dementia. (As I explained earlier, for most of us a 10–12 per cent calorie cut isn't much: the rough equivalent of three chocolate chip cookies or a small portion of McDonald's fries).

As if that weren't enough, the people who took part in this two-year study lost on average 7.5kg – that's 16.5lb, well over a stone – in the process. Those in the control group, on the other hand, very slightly gained weight (0.1kg, or 3.5oz).

The study was called the CALERIE (Comprehensive Assessment

of Long-term Effects of Reduced Intake of Energy) trial.[1]

More than 200 men and women aged between 21 and 50 took part. None of them were clinically obese, but they weren't super slim, either: they had BMIs (body mass index) ranging from 22 to 28. To put this into context, someone who is 170cm (5ft 7in) tall and weighs 70kg (11 stone) has a BMI of 24.

And the health benefits were extraordinary. They included:

- a decrease in 'bad' cholesterol (LDL)
- an increase in 'good' cholesterol (HDL)
- a rapid reduction in blood pressure;
- a profound improvement in insulin sensitivity and reduction in circulating levels of insulin
- a reduction in C-reactive protein (CTP) – high levels of CTP indicate inflammation, especially as an indicator of risk for cardiovascular problems
- improved sleep
- improved mood
- improved libido

Not only that: when researchers did tests for their biological age afterwards,[2] what they found was astonishing. For every chronological year the men and women lived, they had aged biologically by *just one month*.

---

1 Two Years of Calorie Restriction and Cardiometabolic Risk Factors. *Lancet Diabetes Endocrinol.*, 2019 – pmc.ncbi.nlm.nih.gov/articles/PMC6707879/
and
Effect of Calorie Restriction on Mood, Quality of Life, Sleep, and Sexual Function in Healthy Nonobese Adults. *JAMA*, 2017 – jamanetwork.com/journals/jamainternalmedicine/fullarticle/2517920
2 Change in the Rate of Biological Aging in Response to Caloric Restriction. *J. Gerontol. A. Biol. Sci. Med. Sci.*, 2017 – doi: 10.1093/gerona/glx096

Why does caloric restriction have such astonishing health benefits? The answer is quite simple, according to Professor Bill Kraus, whom we met in the last chapter. He has been involved in the CALERIE trial and subsequent research into its findings from the beginning.

'People are overfed. And if you go from being overfed to being normal fed, you see big benefits.' The recommended reduction in calories, Professor Kraus points out, really isn't much: 'It's a scone at Starbucks, right? That's it. You just give that up and you've done it.'

But the beauty of the CALERIE trial is that anyone can adopt the same protocol to achieve these health benefits. The participants didn't eat any sort of special diet: the whole idea, he says, was for them to stick to their usual diet, just with fewer calories.

Because for most people, reducing calories by 30 per cent is an unattainable goal, the CALERIE trial set a slightly lower target of reducing daily food intake by a quarter – 25 per cent – but this also proved too much for most. What the participants did manage – 11.9 per cent, sustained for two years – is a much more realistic target. And it still resulted in incredible benefits.

This plan will show you just how easy it is to make this modest reduction in calories, using two simple but effective methods:

1. **Increasing your fibre.** A high-fibre diet is an effortlessly effective way of cutting your calories – put simply, eating more plants means you feel fuller for longer and so you eat less. It is also extremely good for you: most of us in Britain and the US eat less than half the fibre that we need for optimum health. You'll find this step much easier than you think. All you have to do is follow my Fabulous Fibre plan.

Fibre has for too long been underappreciated, or even ignored. While protein, fats and carbs are the celebrities of the food world, the ones that attract all the passion and attention, fibre is the quiet, uncool one at the back, the one people don't like to talk about – useful, but really, really not glamorous. We think of fibre as just that thing that prevents constipation and keeps our bowels regular. But it does *so* much more than that. It really is the unsung hero of the four major food groups.

In fact, fibre offers many of the same health benefits as caloric restriction. It is the most anti-inflammatory food there is;[3] it improves gut and heart health, blood sugar control and immune function; it lowers 'bad' cholesterol and the risk of several cancers, including colorectal, breast, pancreatic and bladder cancer; and it helps with weight management. A review of more than a dozen international studies[4] showed that increasing fibre by just 14g a day leads to weight loss of 1.9kg (4lb) in less than four months – *without changing anything else that you normally eat.*

How? Because as soon as you increase your fibre intake, you also increase satiety, or how full you feel. As you can see, fibre really is fabulous. However, most of us are not getting nearly enough of it for it to properly do its incredible work. In Britain, the average adult eats just 18g of fibre a day; in the US it's even lower, around 17g a day.[5] That's against a recommended daily amount of 30g. (Our bodies, incidentally, were designed to eat far more even than this – our Paleolithic ancestors consumed between 77 and 120g of fibre every day!).

3 Designing and developing a literature-derived, population-based dietary inflammatory index. *Public Health Nutr.*, 2013 – www.ncbi.nlm.nih.gov/pmc/articles/PMC3925198/
4 Dietary fiber and weight regulation. *Nutr. Rev.*, 2001 – pubmed.ncbi.nlm.nih.gov/11396693/
5 The UK government recommendation is 30g a day. The US government recommendation, meanwhile, for women under 50 is 25g a day (21g a day for those over 50) and 38g a day for men (30g a day for men over 50).

2. Practising a very manageable form of Time Restricted Eating (TRE), where you don't eat anything (or drink anything other than water, black tea, etc) from the time you finish your evening meal until breakfast the next day.

Remember what I said in the previous chapter about having to force our body, ideally every day, into some sort of DIScomfort in order to enable it to go into autophagy, or repair mode? Well, TRE is one of the best ways to do this. It is a mild form of fasting, which involves increasing your overnight fasting window from an average 8–10 hours to 12. You can do this by either eating your last meal of the day earlier or delaying your breakfast, or both.

* * *

Let's first take a closer look at what exactly fibre is, and how it works.

SOLUBLE V INSOLUBLE FIBRE

There are two main types of fibre, soluble and insoluble. Soluble fibre, which is found in foods like peas, beans, apples, bananas and avocados, dissolves in water and forms a gel in the stomach which slows down digestion and helps increase satiety. Insoluble fibre – also known as roughage – doesn't dissolve in water, but it helps the movement of food through the digestive system and adds bulk to stools, meaning it's very helpful for constipation and for keeping bowel movements regular. Examples of insoluble fibre include nuts, green beans, wheat bran and wholewheat flour.

So one consequence of eating more fibre is that you feel fuller more quickly; and as a result, you consume fewer calories – around 10 per cent for most people – hence the weight loss.

According to Dr Michael Greger, who runs a not-for-profit organisation which studies and collates the information from the latest nutritional research globally, 'telling people to increase their intake of fibre-rich foods may actually be one of the single most effective pieces of advice for weight loss'.

Even if you don't want or need to lose weight, you should still eat more fibre. Multiple studies[6] have found that a higher intake of fibre was associated with a 15 per cent lower risk of premature death *from all causes combined.*

FIBRE AND THE MICROBIOME

The reason that fibre is the most anti-inflammatory food you can eat is that it feeds microbes in our gut, which use it to make short-chain fatty acids (SCFAs).

One of these SCFAs is butyrate, which is released into the bloodstream and promotes anti-inflammatory activities throughout the body. How does it do this? Well, partly by enhancing the secretion of a substance called interleukin-10, or IL-10, which is perhaps the most potent anti-inflammatory activator produced by our cells. IL-10 is a cytokine – a type of small protein that

---

6 Eating more fibre linked to reduced risk of non-communicable diseases and death. *BMJ*, 2019 – BMJ 2019;364:l159

and

Association between dietary fiber and lower risk of all-cause mortality: a meta-analysis of cohort studies. *Am. J. Epidemiol.* 2015 – doi: 10.1093/aje/kwu257 circulates through our blood and helps regulate our immune response, preventing it from overreacting.

This may explain, adds Dr Greger, why people who eat fibre-rich foods are less likely to develop inflammatory conditions, from knee pain to osteoarthritis, to lung inflammation, respiratory diseases and cancer.

A 2024 review in the journal *Nature*[7] found that the association between a high-dietary-fibre intake and lower incidence of colorectal and breast cancer has been consistently reported, and notes that meta-analyses (which look at many studies to establish overall patterns) have also reported a similar link between high-fibre diets and lower incidence of pancreatic, bladder, ovarian and endometrial cancers. The review noted that butyrate is particularly beneficial in this process.

SFCAs even cross from the blood into the brain, enhancing its overall health and development.[8] So far, all studies have been done in rats and mice, but have consistently shown that SCFAs improve recovery from stroke; and also help to alleviate depression, decrease stress in the central nervous system, reduce neuro-inflammation and even improve memory.

SCFAs like butyrate also stimulate production of leptin, a hormone that sends a signal to our brain telling us we need to eat less.

---

7 The gut microbiome and dietary fibres: implications in obesity, cardiometabolic diseases and cancer. *Nature*, 2024 – www.nature.com/articles/s41579-024-01108-z
8 The role of short-chain fatty acids from gut microbiota in gut-brain communication. *Front. Endocrinol.*, 2020 – www.frontiersin.org/journals/endocrinology/articles/10.3389/fendo.2020.00025/full
and
Gut microbiotic features aiding the diagnosis of acute ischemic stroke, *Front. Cell. Infect. Microbiol.*, 2020 – doi: 10.3389/fcimb.2020.587284

THE POWER OF PLANTS

The other great thing about fibre is that it is only found in plants, and consequently, eating it increases your intake of three crucial macronutrients that combine to provide truly astonishing health and longevity benefits: **plant protein** (beans, peas, lentils, nuts), **complex carbohydrates** (beans, peas and lentils again, together with wholegrains and fibre-rich vegetables such as broccoli, carrots, sweet potatoes, apples, pears), and **healthy fats** (nuts and olive oil).

Plant protein

Like carbohydrates and fats, protein gives us energy. When we digest protein from our food, it is broken down into amino acids, which the body then uses to build all the thousands of different proteins it needs to do everything from keeping our muscles and bones healthy to supporting our immune system.

Meat, dairy, eggs and fish are all good sources of protein. But it's plant protein that appears to offer the most longevity benefits (see more on protein on p65).

How to get plant protein? Easy – eat more beans, peas and lentils. These are excellent sources and like all protein will increase your satiety.

Unlike protein from meat, however, they also decrease cholesterol and blood pressure – as one 2023 study of identical twins showed,[9] in as little as eight weeks.

I'm not saying don't eat meat – far from it, please carry on if you enjoy it (which I certainly do). I'm just suggesting that you cut down, and swap some of the meat you usually eat for plant protein instead.

9 Cardiometabolic effects of omnivorous vs vegan diets in identical twins. *JAMA Netw Open*, 2023 – jamanetwork.com/journals/jamanetworkopen/fullarticle/2812392

Complex carbohydrates

Complex carbohydrates are foods that release their energy slowly. They contain longer chains of sugar molecules than simple carbs and take longer to digest. As a result, they fuel our bodies slowly and consistently and keep us fuller for longer. Common examples of complex carbs are legumes, such as beans, peas and lentils; starchy vegetables, such as potatoes, parsnips, carrots; and wholegrain foods like brown rice, oatmeal and quinoa.

Complex carbohydrates are mostly unrefined – that is to say, in their natural state; for example, wholegrain bread and pasta and brown or wild rice rather than the white versions.

By contrast, refined, or simple carbs (sometimes referred to as 'bad' carbs) are something you should avoid, where possible. They include refined grains that have been stripped of all fibre and nutrients, such as white bread, pizza dough, pasta, pastries, white flour, white rice and many breakfast cereals; sugary treats, such as cakes and biscuits; as well as foods previously thought of as 'healthy', like fruit juice and honey.

Healthy fats

Healthy, unsaturated fats are crucial for all aspects of our health, including our brain health. These include olive oil, nuts – especially walnuts, which are high in a type of omega-3 fatty acid called alpha-linolenic acid (ALA) that helps lower blood pressure and protect arteries – fish such as cod and salmon, and avocados.

Saturated fats, on the other hand, which are found naturally in animal products – meat, cheese, butter – have been associated with a higher risk of cardiovascular disease, because they increase 'bad' cholesterol. And when food contains both sugar and saturated fats, which is the case in many ultra-processed products, the combination becomes really deleterious to human health: obesity, blocked arteries and even reduced memory. In one study,[10] people who ate a diet comprised mostly of roast meat, sausages, hamburgers, steak, chips, crisps and soft drinks saw significantly more shrinkage in their hippocampus (a key memory centre in the brain) than those eating healthy diets.

So it is best to lower your consumption of dairy products and meat and, when you do eat meat, try to grill or boil it rather than fry it. Frying or roasting meat in oil at high temperatures causes a chemical reaction known as glycation, which is implicated in inflammatory and lifestyle disorders like diabetes, athero-sclerosis, cardiovascular diseases and rheumatoid arthritis, as well as Alzheimer's disease, cataracts and cancer.[11] Food that is highly processed – as in ready-made pastries, cakes, biscuits and crisps, for example – is also highly glycated, so best avoided.

Again, I'm not asking you to give up cake. That way madness lies (for me at least), as a world without cake is miserable indeed. But what you can do is start making it a habit to reach for a handful of nuts whenever you want a snack in order to reduce your dependency on sugar and saturated fat. Then, when you do have some cake or a couple of biscuits, the impact on your body will be far less, particularly if you make your own (and especially if you swap the butter for olive oil whenever possible).

Similarly, make it a habit to choose hard cheese (for example, Gruyere, Cheddar, Manchego) rather than soft, as soft cheeses (for example, Camembert, ricotta, Brie) have more saturated fat. A couple of rye crackers with Gruyere or Manchego make a

---

10. Western diet is associated with a smaller hippocampus. *BMC Med.*, 2015 – doi: 10.1186/s12916-015-0461-x
11 Increased advanced glycation end product specific fluorescence in repeatedly heated used cooking oil. *J. Food Science & Tech.*, 2017 – doi: 10.1007/s13197-017-2682-9

tasty, filling snack and are much better for you than French bread with Brie.

A note on olive oil … You might wonder why this tends to be the only oil described as a healthy fat – what about other plant-based varieties, such as vegetable oil or sunflower oil? The answer is to do with processing. Most vegetable oil is made from a mixture of canola, sunflower, soybean or corn, and so more processing is required to remove impurities and create a neutral flavoured blend. This affects its nutritional value, making it higher in omega-6, which is pro-inflammatory and not good for us in high doses. Olive oil, on the other hand, especially extra virgin, is among the least processed cooking oils, which means it retains the most antioxidants, vitamins and minerals. I can't stress enough how good olive oil is for you. Invest in the best quality you can afford. Cook with it, drizzle it on vegetables and salads, and if you're really keen, drink an extra tablespoon a day neat. (Bryan Johnson says the second-best thing you can do for your longevity – the first being getting enough sleep every single night – is to have three tablespoons of top-quality extra-virgin olive oil a day: its combination of fatty acids and polyphenols reduces inflammation and 'bad' LDL cholesterol, increases 'good' HDL cholesterol and lowers blood pressure. One US study[12] showed regular consumption reduces your chances of dying from any cause by almost a fifth (19 per cent).

* * *

---

12 Consumption of olive oil and risk of total and cause-specific mortality among US adults. *J Am Coll Cardiol.*, 2022 –pmc.ncbi.nlm.nih.gov/articles/PMC8851878/pdf/nihms-1758221.pdf

As for TRE, the mild form I am advocating – with 12-hour overnight fasts – really is relatively easy to sustain. Obviously, you can't do it every day – you need to be able to have a late dinner here and there, or go to a party when you want to! But on ordinary days at home, it simply means having no snacks or treats after your evening meal. It is extremely good for your health, and it is safe, unlike other methods of fasting, such as intermittent fasting, or TRE with longer periods of abstinence such as 16 hours. Those methods carry the risk of potentially dangerous side effects, as many people find the easiest way to sustain these regimes is by not eating breakfast – and there is growing evidence that skipping breakfast is not a good idea.

In 2024, there was much controversy around a study from Shanghai Jiao Tong University[13] claiming that people who limited their eating window to less than eight hours a day, fasting for the other 16 hours, doubled their risk of dying from cardiovascular diseases compared to those who fasted only 8–12 hours.

Many experts pointed out that the study was flawed. The participants self-reported their food intake (people are notoriously unreliable when it comes to saying what they've eaten); and the data, although covering 20,000 people over eight years, relied on them detailing what they ate over just two days. There was no information on what, and when, they'd eaten for the rest of the time.

However, other, more reliable studies have shown the same worrying effect, including an increased risk of cardiovascular disease in people who skip breakfast.

---

13 8-hour time-restricted eating linked to a 91% higher risk of cardiovascular death *Science Daily*, 2024 – www.sciencedaily.com/releases/2024/03/240320115727.htm

Two recent studies – one published in *Nature Communications* in 2023[14] of data from more than 100,000 people, the other, a 2020 meta-analysis published in the *Journal of Clinical Nutrition*[15] of seven studies involving 220,000 people – have confirmed findings from multiple previous studies that skipping breakfast increases the risk of cardiovascular disease. The first found that the risk is higher for women; the second, that skipping breakfast not only increases the risk of cardiovascular disease, but also of dying from any cause.

None of this is definitive, of course. But it needs to be taken into account when you decide how you want to go about eating less often. It's the reason Valter Longo advises doing TRE with just a 12-hour fasting window – for example, eating no food after 7pm or 8pm and not eating again until 7am or 8am.

Professor Kraus gives similar advice to his cardiac patients. 'I tell my patients – do not eat after dinner. The first question I ask them about their lifestyle is, "Do you eat after dinner?" And if I can get them to stop eating after dinner, that's probably at least a 10-hour fast.'

Here then are the headlines: over the next three weeks your primary goal is to eat a little bit less than you do now. Moving to a higher-fibre diet alone will make a huge difference to your health. It will not only improve everything from your cardiovascular health to your risk of diabetes and cancer, it will also naturally reduce your caloric intake by that magic 10–12 per cent we're aiming for – a caloric restriction which is doable, sustainable and can even

---

14 Dietary circadian rhythms and cardiovascular disease risk in the prospective NutriNet-Santé cohort. *Nat. Commun.*, 2023 – doi.org/10.1038/s41467-023-43444-3
15 Association between skipping breakfast and risk of cardiovascular disease and all cause mortality. *Clin. Nutr.*, 2020 – doi.org/10.1016/j,clnu.2020.02.004

reduce your biological age.

By eating more fibre, you'll naturally find you are eating more plant protein and complex carbs, while also eating fewer unhealthy saturated fats, partly because you'll be trying actively to avoid them and partly because you'll be so full.

You'll feel less in need of sugary snacks. You'll start to have more energy. And you may well find you weigh a little less.

Add in the very mildest form of TRE, by leaving a minimum of 12 hours between your last meal of the day and your first meal the next day, and in longevity terms you will be well and truly launched.

The way I do TRE

For me, I find what works best is a 14-hour window: no food after 8.30 or 9pm, and none the next day before 10.30 or 11am. That's when I have breakfast (at my desk, usually), so that I'm not skipping it, just eating it later than the usual time.

This timeframe happens to suit me because for as long as I can remember, I've had no desire to eat breakfast first thing. I'm simply not hungry until 10 or 11am. I exercise early in the morning and prefer to do so on an empty stomach: again, that just suits my body best. But even in the many years when I wasn't exercising, I still wasn't hungry before mid-morning.

I urge you to find the timeframe that makes your body feel its best and which also fits in with your lifestyle, depending on the shape of your day.

What is clear from many studies is that people find TRE the easiest kind of regular fasting to maintain consistently. And, as consistency is the most important factor, it's worth doing for that reason alone.

GO GENTLY

Of course, when it comes to increasing your fibre intake, it's not wise to make all these changes at once. If you switch overnight from a diet low in fibre and high in saturated fat to one that is high in fibre and low in saturated fat, your body will struggle to process such a drastic and sudden change. You may well have some physical reactions – bloating or constipation – and probably decide to give up. Game over before it's really begun.

Likewise, it will take time to embrace TRE. If you have been used to having dinner late, or having it early and then topping up with a late-night snack, you may feel quite disorientated to start with as you face the apparently long evening ahead.

This is where the plan comes in. It's a friendly, gentle guide to help you make the changes *gradually*, allowing your body and your mind time to comfortably adjust.

I really encourage you to commit to the Fabulous Fibre/TRE diet for three weeks. I know it's hard to be motivated, especially when it comes to eating beans – I spent decades not so much avoiding them as never even thinking about them. Now, though, I love them.

What I can promise is that you will feel better within this short time. And you may find that it gives you all the motivation you need to keep going.

So what are you waiting for? Let's go!

EATING LESS:
The three-week reset

First, a quiz.

The multiple choice questions below are designed to help you learn more about how healthily you eat now. Then, armed with that information, you can start the three-week programme. It isn't as hard as you think – and just remember, according to David Sinclair and Valter Longo, two of the most pre-eminent longevity scientists in the world today, it is the single most important thing you can do to live longer in good health.

1 **How many different vegetables do you eat a day?**
  a. 0–2
  b. 3–5
  c. 5–7
  d. Just call me Gwynnie...

2 **What sort of protein (meat, cheese, eggs, beans, nuts) do you eat on a typical day?**
  a. A burger, fried chicken
  b. Spaghetti bolognese, bacon and egg or sausages and baked beans
  c. 50g of lean chicken or turkey, occasionally a good steak, some cheese and a handful of nuts
  d. Tofu, Greek yoghurt, black bean stew

③ Which sort of carbs do you eat on a typical day?
    a. Toast, sausage roll, cake, macaroni cheese
    b. Breakfast cereal, cheese sandwich, crisps, chicken pie and mash
    c. Bread for lunchtime sandwich, the occasional pasta for dinner
    d. Bulgur wheat, leafy green vegetables, dark chocolate as a treat

④ How many sweet foods and snacks do you eat on a typical day?
    a. Toast or croissant with jam or honey, or cereal at breakfast; chocolate biscuits or cake mid-morning; pastry at teatime; pudding after dinner.
    b. Yoghurt and granola with berry compote; apple for mid-morning snack; pudding after dinner.
    c. Wholemeal toast with organic honey for breakfast; nuts for afternoon snack; dinner followed by cheese and grapes.
    d. Cheese and tomato on rye crackers or a handful of almonds for afternoon snack; two squares of dark chocolate with raspberries after dinner.

⑤ How many meals do you eat a day?
    a. Breakfast, morning snack, lunch, afternoon snack, dinner, pudding, late-night snack
    b. Breakfast, lunch, afternoon snack, dinner with dessert
    c. Breakfast, lunch, afternoon snack, late dinner
    d. Breakfast, light lunch, large early dinner, with occasional snacks.

Scores
Mostly a: Complete beginner. Don't worry. This programme is designed to be easy to follow and you will find you can do it perfectly well.

Mostly b: Intermediate. You are already making some healthy choices on the road to longevity. This programme will help move you further along. If you want to try one or two of the challenges along the way, that's fine.

Mostly c: Advanced. You are doing really well. This programme will optimise your longevity potential – take on the extra challenges whenever you can, as you are certainly ready for them.

Mostly d: Valter Longo level – you're on your way to living to 120! If you are not doing so already, think about doing the five-day fast, as recommended by Dr Longo, two or three times a year.

* * *

Here's how the plan works. Over the next three weeks, you are going to increase your fibre intake; and you're going to gradually introduce some TRE.

To help you do this, I give some general principles to follow, as to what to eat and what to avoid –as well as a list of high-fibre foods (some of these are surprising!) and lots of tips and advice on how to incorporate these into your daily meals.

In addition, I provide plenty of examples of each of the four macronutrients – fibre, plant protein, complex carbs and unsaturated fats – to show you how to get the maximum longevity bang for your health buck.

And finally, I offer three weeks of sample menus, which include simple meal suggestions and show you how to make a gentle transition that allows both your body and your mind to acclimatise to this new way of eating.

You do not need to follow my menus, of course. If you are a confident cook, you may want to devise your own. But whether you are following my menus or going it alone, I urge you to familiarise yourself with what you are eating in advance and make a careful shopping list so you are well prepared. The key when trying to stick to a new eating plan is to minimise the risk of having to make a last-minute dash for something instant from the local shop.

WEEK 1

Aim: to have a fibre-rich breakfast containing at least 8g of fibre for five days this week, and, on one day, to introduce a 12-hour fasting window – for example, eating no food after 7pm or 8pm and not eating again until 7am or 8am.

We are building up to 30g of fibre a day gradually, so in this first week, we'll focus only on breakfast, aiming for it to include a minimum of 8g. (As I mentioned before, it is not a good idea to skip breakfast so do try to have it.)

Fab fibre tip 1

Drink more water, particularly before a meal. Not only does this help move the fibre through your system, but research shows that drinking two glasses of water 30 minutes before you eat a meal results in consuming around 20 per cent fewer calories.[1]

---

1 Immediate pre-meal water ingestion decreases voluntary food intake in lean young males. *Eur. J. Nutr.*, 2016 – pubmed.ncbi.nlm.nih. gov/25893719/

WEEK 2

Aim: to have a fibre-rich lunch containing a minimum of 10g of fibre on at least four days this week and continuing with the fibre-rich breakfast on five days. Also, increase your TRE to include a 12-hour fasting window on two days.

By the end of the second week you will be well on your way to the target of 30g fibre a day and getting the hang of TRE.

WEEK 3

Aim: to include a minimum of 10g of fibre in your evening meal on at least three days (continuing the fibre-rich breakfast on five days and lunch on four days as well), and to practise TRE on three days – you can choose whether to do this on your high-fibre days or not.

So there you have it: simple! Over the course of three weeks, you are aiming to increase your daily fibre intake by eating more delicious and healthy plant foods, and to give your body a little more precious down time overnight to allow it to go into repair mode.

Fab fibre tip 2

As well as drinking more, move more too. This will help you to avoid constipation and bloating.

FOODS THAT ARE HIGH IN FIBRE

(Listed with highest-fibre food first and based on average serving size of each food)

- 1 avocado 10g
- 100g rolled oats, raw 10g; cooked 1.7g
- 150g punnet of raspberries 8g

120g (= half a 400g can, drained) butter beans 8g

120g (= half a 400g can, drained) chickpeas 8g

100g lentils, cooked 7.9g

1 medium (175g) jacket potato 5.8g

100g peas boiled 5.5g

1 medium pear, skin on 5.5g

100g broad beans, boiled 5.4g

200g sweet potato, baked, without skin 5g

1 medium apple, skin on 4.4g

Wholewheat English muffin (66g) 4.4g

400g tin chopped tomatoes 4g

Half a tin (207g) Heinz baked beans 3.9g

175g Swiss chard, cooked 3.7g

100g wholewheat pasta 3.6g

150g cauliflower (about one quarter), cooked 3.5g

1 slice wholemeal bread 3.5g

100g new potatoes, skin on 3.3g

100g French green beans, cooked 3.2 g

100g kalamata olives, pitted 3.2g

1 banana 3.1g

140g tin Green Giant organic sweetcorn, drained 3g

1 slice multigrain bread 3g

100g quinoa, cooked 2.8g

1 tbsp flaxseed 2.8g

25g almonds 2.7g

100g aubergine (1 aubergine is approx. 250–300g), cooked 2.5g

1 homemade Greek flatbread made with Greek yoghurt mixed with half wholemeal flour, half self-raising 2.5g

1 medium carrot (approx. 80g) 2.4g

100g broccoli (approx. 7 stems), steamed 2.4g

100g spinach, cooked, 2.4g

100g mushrooms (4 baby portobello mushrooms), cooked 2.2g

100g (= approx. half) red onion 2.2g

100g cherry tomatoes (6–10 depending on size) 2g

100g green olives 1.9g

100g leek, cooked 1.8g

100g wild rice, cooked 1.8g (compared to 0.4g for 100g white rice, cooked)

100g brown rice, cooked 1.6g

25g walnuts 1.3g

100g celeriac, boiled 1.2g

100g (= approx. half) white onion 1.2g

1 tbsp sesame seeds 1.1g

100g courgette, cooked 1g

1 tbsp pumpkin seeds 1g

1 tbsp peanut butter 1g

1 tbsp hummus 0.8g

100g cucumber, peel on 0.7g

100g watercress 0.5g

Sources: United States Department of Agriculture FoodData Central/MyFoodData.com/brand where named

Examples of plants high in protein
Chickpeas
Butter beans
Black beans
Lentils
Peas

In the UK, the government recommended daily minimum for protein is 45g for women, 55.5g for men (adults aged 19–64).

Examples of complex carbohydrates
Wholegrain bread
Wholewheat pasta
Bulgur wheat
Brown or wild rice
Starchy vegetables (sweet potatoes, corn, peas)
Legumes: black beans, kidney beans, lentils, butter beans

In the UK, the government recommended daily minimum for carbs is 267g for women, 333g for men. That is actually a lot of carbs: there are 12g of carbs in one slice of multigrain bread; 45g in two medium sweet potatoes; 45g in one cup of cooked long grain rice; almost 18g in half a can of butter beans.

Examples of foods high in unsaturated fats
Oils from single vegetables and nuts, for example olive oil, sunflower oil, walnut oil, sesame oil
Nuts, especially almonds, cashews, pecans, peanuts, walnuts, and seeds: pumpkin seeds, sesame seeds, flaxseed
Avocados
Oily fish such as salmon, mackerel, herring, anchovies or tuna

The UK government guidelines for adult fat intake are 97g per day for men and 78g per day for women, most of which should be unsaturated – less than a third (31g men; 24g women) should be saturated.

HEALTHY FOOD HACKS

- Swap white pasta for wholewheat, and replace half of your pasta portion with lentils, or any sort of bean.
- Choose multigrain or dark seeded rye bread rather than white.
- Swap half the meat in any dish for butterbeans, chickpeas or lentils.
- Choose peanut or other nut butter instead of butter and jam.
- Make a delicious alternative to cake by smearing an oatcake with nut butter and honey.
- Try and keep croissants, pastries, etc, for a special treat. If you are used to having a croissant for breakfast, go for the ones with a savoury protein filling, such as cheese or ham, which will help mitigate the glucose spike that occurs whenever you eat something sweet on an empty stomach (but bear in mind that a croissant still counts as an ultra-processed food, and along with the sugar you're also getting a dose of saturated fat – plus a high number of calories that won't help in your quest to eat 10 per cent less!).
- If you like something sweet for breakfast, try plain Greek yoghurt with nuts and berries. (Or you could follow Dr Longo's example. He eats an Italian hard bread called friselle for breakfast, together with a spread made from almonds and cocoa, followed by an apple.)

- All berries are good, but note that raspberries have three times as much fibre (7g fibre per 100g) as blueberries.
- Eat more fatty fish like salmon and cod. Limit tuna consumption to avoid mercury poisoning.
- Scatter pumpkin seeds, sesame seeds or sunflower seeds over vegetables or in a salad.
- Ditch the peeler! Keep the skin on potatoes, apples, pears and as many other fruits and veg as possible.
- If you love chocolate, have some! Just try to go for dark chocolate, and keep it as a treat for after your main meal of the day. (If you love milk chocolate, slowly replace it, block by block if need be, with a darker variety, gradually increasing the cocoa content. I've got myself up to 75 per cent cocoa content like this; Dr Longo says he is now up to 85 per cent).

WHAT NOT TO EAT

Ultra-processed food

According to one study quoted by Dr Chris van Tulleken, who studies the food industry and its effects on our health, up to 60 per cent of the average UK diet is made up of ultra-processed food, or UPF. Which is very scary, because UPF not only makes us fat, it is also strongly associated with an increased risk of stroke, heart attack, cancer, type 2 diabetes, irritable bowel syndrome, high blood pressure and depression.

What is UPF, exactly? The definition given by Dr van Tulleken in his book *Ultra Processed People* (which I highly recommend for its terrifying insight into exactly what ultra-processed food is and what it does to us) is any food which is 'wrapped in plastic and which contains at least one ingredient you wouldn't usually find in a standard home kitchen'.

Much of it is what we know as junk food – but not just junk food. 'There's plenty of organic, free range, "ethical" UPF too,' he says. 'It's a rule of thumb that almost every food that comes with a health claim on the packet is a UPF.'

Ultra-processed food as an idea was first suggested in 2010 by a Brazilian professor of nutrition, Carlos Monteiro, who put forward the theory that UPF was responsible for the rapid rise in obesity.

He defined UPFs as involving 'the fractioning of whole foods into substances and chemical modifications of those substances…', adding that the 'processes and ingredients used to manufacture ultra-processed foods are designed to create highly profitable (low-cost ingredients, long shelf life, emphatic branding) convenient (ready to consume) hyperplatable products liable to displace freshly prepared dishes and meals…'

Professor Monteiro's theory was put to the test in a study conducted by Kevin Hall, senior investigator at the US National Institute of Diabetes and Digestive and Kidney Diseases. In the study, two groups of volunteers were given identical diets in terms of how much fat, salt, sugar and fibre they contained, but one diet was made up of UPF, and the other of unprocessed food. They were all allowed to eat as much as they wanted.

All the volunteers on the UPF diet put on weight, while all the volunteers on the unprocessed food diet lost weight. When the researchers assessed the results, they discovered that on average people on the UPF diet consumed 500 more calories a day than those on the unprocessed food diet.

When he was writing his book, Dr van Tulleken put himself on a UPF diet for a month to see what happened. In just four weeks he put on 6kg, increased his markers for inflammation and totally derailed his appetite hormones: 'The hormone that signals fullness barely responded after a large meal, while the hunger hormone was sky high just moments after eating.'

Sugar

Aside from the fact that eating too much of it can lead to diabetes, sugar activates two genes, RAS and PKA, that are known to accelerate ageing (this groundbreaking discovery was made more than 20 years ago by Dr Longo, together with the fact that starving yeast organisms of everything but water made them live twice as long. It was an astonishing longevity breakthrough – he had not only identified one of the first genes regulating the ageing process, but also the entire signalling pathway and connection with food.)

So you should be aiming to eat a low-sugar diet, which means avoiding not only sweets and desserts but also refined carbohydrates such as pasta, white bread and rice (which convert easily into sugar).

Many of us don't realise just how much sugar there is in white rice, potatoes and bread. The teaspoon of sugar you have a few times a day in your tea or coffee may amount to far less, once it's processed in your bloodstream, than the sugar you consume from a large helping of white rice or mashed potato.

Here's the good news, though: fibre naturally helps improve blood sugar control because it slows down the absorption of food, including any sugar that's in it, leading to fewer blood sugar spikes and therefore fewer sugar cravings (which are the result of the drop in blood sugar that follows a spike, as what goes up must also come down!). This is especially true of soluble fibre. So if, like me, you can't get through the day without at least a little chocolate, your increased fibre intake will reduce its impact.

At the same time, once you're eating more fibre and unrefined carbs, you'll find it much easier to cut down on sweet treats, because as I've explained, fibre-rich foods are incredibly filling. You won't crave sugary foods nearly as much and when you do eat something with natural sugars – such as a strawberry, orange or tomato – you'll be astonished at the explosion of sweetness.

THE LOWDOWN ON PROTEIN

It was Dr Longo's research (again) that provided a key longevity insight into protein. He has spent years studying a group of people in Ecuador with defects in the growth hormone receptor gene. This makes them rather short in terms of stature but big in terms of survival, as they rarely develop diabetes or cancer, have a reduced incidence of other diseases and also appear to have more youthful brain function.

High protein intake, he explains, causes the activation of the growth hormone receptor, which in turn increases the levels of insulin and insulin-like growth factor (IGF-1) – higher levels of both of which are associated with diabetes and cancer. In addition, proteins can activate TOR-S6K, genes that accelerate ageing, and whose role in ageing his lab discovered, as reported in *Science* in 2001.[16] (You may remember that he also discovered that the gene PKA, activated by sugar, also plays a key role in ageing).

He concluded that reducing calorie intake, particularly by reducing calories from proteins and sugars, decreases growth

---

16 Regulation of Longevity and Stress Resistance by Sch9 in Yeast: Rising to the challenges of old age. *Science*, 2001 – www.science.org/doi/10.5555/ sageke.2001.1.or3

hormone receptor activity and therefore the TOR-S6K and PKA genes known to accelerate ageing.

The TOR-S6K pathway went on to be shown by many laboratories to be perhaps the most potent set of genes to accelerate ageing. In a famous 2009 paper published in *Nature*,[17] three US laboratories showed that inhibiting TOR-S6K signalling with the drug rapamycin extended lifespan and healthspan in mice.

So Dr Longo recommends keeping protein intake sufficient but low, as well as getting the bulk of what protein you do eat from plants, nuts and fish rather than meat or dairy.

Many experts, including Michael Greger, Tim Spector and David Sinclair (who recently changed to an entirely vegan diet) make the same recommendations.

As David Sinclair says, 'This doesn't mean a little red meat will kill you, but when we substitute animal protein with more plant protein, studies have shown that all-cause mortality falls significantly.'

Tim Spector points out that many studies have shown that on average vegans and vegetarians are healthier and live longer in most countries. In addition, he says, people who eat meat also tend to have fewer 'good' microbiome species – the microbiome being the different bacteria we all have in our guts. A good microbiome helps reduce chronic inflammation, which is associated with nearly every long-term disease we can think of.

But Dr Peter Attia, another highly respected longevity expert, disagrees. He thinks we need more protein rather than less, and strongly believes that the protein we get from animals – such as meat, eggs and cheese – is better for us. (Longo, by the way,

---

17 Rapamycin fed late in life extends lifespan in genetically heterogeneous mice. *Nature*, 2009 – https://www.nature.com/articles/nature08221

wholeheartedly disagrees! He says there is very little evidence for this, and overwhelming evidence against it when you look at epidemiological, clinical mouse and centenarian studies.)

What they all agree on is that older people – those aged 65 and above – definitely need more protein, because as we get older we lose muscle mass and process protein less effectively.

SAMPLE MENUS

The meal plans on the next few pages are just an illustration to give you a rough guide to what it takes to achieve a high-fibre diet. Remember that you are going slowly to give your gut a chance to acclimatise – starting with a high-fibre breakfast on five days in week 1, adding in a fibre-rich lunch on four days in week 2, and finally adding more fibre to your evening meal on at least three days in week 3 (keeping the fibre-rich breakfast on five days and lunch on four days as well).

I've offered a good variety of simple healthy and tasty meals, and given approximate fibre counts for each (for one serving). If you were to eat all the meals in this plan with the fibre quantities shown, by week three you'd be eating 32–40g of fibre a day.

I've deliberately given no quantities other than for fibre, as the amount I eat and require for my individual needs (I'm 5ft 5in/165cm and 8st 11lb/56kg) may be very different from yours, especially if you are taller, heavier or more active than me. I've also not included snacks or puddings, which of course you will probably have at least some of the time – as do I.

WEEK 1: BREAKFAST

Choose from the following breakfast options on five days this week. Remember to drink at least a glass of water either before or with each breakfast.

Slice multigrain bread with **at least 1 tbsp peanut butter** and **a sliced pear. Total fibre: 9.5g**

Plain Greek yoghurt with **at least 100g raspberries** (two-thirds of a punnet) and **25g almonds. Total fibre: 8g**

Slice multigrain bread with scrambled eggs and **at least 200g spinach** and **100g grilled tomatoes. Total fibre: 10g**

Porridge or rolled oats (at least 100g,) cooked with milk with **a minimum of 30g walnuts, 100g raspberries** (two-thirds of a punnet), 1 tsp honey, and cinnamon. **Total fibre: 8.3g**

Poached egg/s with **2 slices multigrain bread,** with **at least 100g broccoli,** steamed and **100g grilled mushrooms. Total fibre: 10.6g**

Wholewheat English muffin with **at least 1 tbsp peanut butter** and **a banana. Total fibre: 8.5g**

At least 2 slices wholemeal toast with **at least 2 tbsp hummus** (you can add dukkah or any other herbs or spice of your choice). **Total fibre: 8.6g**

Note: if you sprinkle **a tbsp of toasted pumpkin seeds** on any of these options, you'll increase your fibre intake even more.

WEEK 2: LUNCH

Sticking to your new breakfasts, choose four from the following lunch options, and try to finish each with an unpeeled apple or pear. This is important as it increases the fibre intake and also means you will be much better able to resist the temptation of cake or biscuits mid-afternoon. Remember: drink at least a glass of water either before or with each meal.

Salad of **tinned chickpeas (minimum 100g, drained weight), green beans (minimum 100g), tomatoes (minimum 100g) and kalamata olives (at least 50g, pitted)** with a Dijon mustard, olive oil and lemon juice dressing. **Total fibre: 11g**

Jacket potato with baked beans (at least 200g) and sweetcorn (at least 100g). Total fibre: 13.7g

Salad of **tinned butter beans (at least 100g, drained weight), green olives (at least 50g), cherry tomatoes (at least 100g), flat-leaf parsley (10g),** with an olive oil and red wine vinegar dressing, and **at least 1 slice wholegrain crusty bread (50g). Total fibre: 13.8g**

Lentil and tomato soup, made with **at least 30g (dry weight) lentils = 80g cooked, 200g tin chopped tomatoes, 1 small onion,** garlic and vegetable stock, and **2 slices crusty wholegrain bread (100g). Total fibre: 17.3g**

Wholewheat pasta (at least 50g, dry weight) with 1 tbsp pesto, **peas (50g), broad beans (50g) and cherry tomatoes (50g)** and 1 tbsp grated Parmesan, with **1 slice crusty wholegrain bread (50g). Total fibre: 16g**

Bruschetta (minimum 2 slices toasted ciabatta bread) **with tomatoes (minimum 100g)** roasted in olive oil and **1 avocado, sliced. Total fibre: 13.6g**

2 slices wholemeal bread with smoked salmon dressed with lemon juice and black pepper, sour cream and dill, **100g steamed broccoli** drizzled with olive oil and lemon juice and sprinkled with **1 tbsp sesame seeds. Total fibre: 10.5g**

LIFELINE: if at all possible, have a short walk – 10 minutes is fine – after lunch. This not only aids digestion and helps control blood sugar, but leaves you calmer and more alert as you go into the afternoon.

WEEK 3: DINNER
Choose three of the following options, to add to your high-fibre breakfast and lunches.

Wholewheat spaghetti (75g, dry weight) with sautéed mushrooms (100g), leeks (100g), spinach (100g), cherry tomatoes (100g), garlic and 1 tbsp grated Parmesan. **Total fibre: 11.4g**

Grilled chicken breast (170g), cooked with lemon and rosemary, new potatoes (100g) skin on, roasted in 1 tbsp olive oil, baked leeks (100g) and a salad of chickpeas (50g, drained weight), raw cauliflower florets (50g) and tomatoes (50g) dressed with olive oil and vinegar, or some Dijon mayonnaise, plus 1 slice crusty wholegrain bread (50g). **Total fibre: 11.3g**

Brown rice (50g, dry weight) lemon pilaf (soak the rice in cold water for 20 minutes; fry half an onion in olive oil in an ovenproof pan, add the drained rice and stir for a minute, then add the juice and zest of half a lemon and 250ml vegetable stock; season, cover and put in a medium oven for 15 minutes or until the rice is cooked and the water has disappeared). Serve with 25g toasted almonds, fresh coriander, 175g Swiss chard, Greek full-fat plain yoghurt and 2 homemade Greek flatbreads (couldn't be easier – mix 70g wholemeal flour with 70g self-raising flour, add 2tsp baking powder and 220g plain Greek yoghurt, knead into a dough, rest half an hour then divide into 4 pieces and roll each one out to a thin circle. Cook on a hot metal skillet. Makes 4. Delicious.). **Total fibre: 13g**

Baked salmon (200g) with 2 tbsp pesto, **50g wild rice (= 150g cooked), 100g steamed green beans, 100g tomatoes, roasted** in olive oil, and **100g steamed peas. Total fibre: 13.4g**

Roast cod (200g) with **lentils (50g, dry weight)**, 2 tbsp salsa verde, **100g steamed broccoli** and **100g tomatoes, roasted** in olive oil. **Total fibre: 12.3g**

Vegetable curry made with **1 medium sweet potato, half a carrot, quarter of a medium cauliflower (approx. 150g), half tin chopped tomatoes, half an onion,** curry powder, 2 tbsp olive oil, **50g frozen peas,** served with 2 tbsp plain yoghurt, **mango chutney** and **50g dry (150g cooked) brown rice. Total fibre: 15.3g**

Bean, pasta and vegetable stew. Fry **half a red onion, at least 50g tomatoes, 100g mushrooms** and **100g courgette** (feel free to substitute vegetables of your choice) with some garlic and fennel seeds in olive oil, then add **at least 120g tinned beans (drained weight)** – cannellini, borlotti and butter beans all work really well; plus **wholewheat pasta (30g, dry weight)** – rigatoni or penne are both good options; and approx. 120ml vegetable stock. Simmer until all ingredients are melded and serve with lots of Parmesan. **Total fibre: 16g**

Fab fibre tip 3

If you ate every one of these meals over seven days you would consume 32 different vegetables, fruits, nuts, seeds and herbs. Research shows that eating 30 different plant types every week is extremely beneficial to the gut microbiome.

VEGETABLE AND FRUIT CHALLENGE

Most of us eat just a few of the same vegetables and fruit week in, week out. It's so easy to get stuck in a rut. Here's how to break out of it.

Using the lists below, make a note of the fruits and vegetables that you eat frequently – for example, tomatoes, potatoes, cucumber, carrots, apples, bananas – and then challenge yourself to try five different ones every week for the next few weeks.

But each week the new additions should be a different five – so that by the end of three weeks you've tried 15 new fruits and veg and hopefully found some new favourites.

Vegetables:

Artichoke, asparagus, aubergine, avocado, beetroot, broccoli, Brussels sprouts, butternut squash, carrot, cauliflower, green cabbage, celery, chicory, collard greens, corn, courgette, cucumber, endive, fennel, green beans, kale, kohlrabi, leek, lettuce, mushrooms, okra, olive, onion, parsnip, peas, potato, pumpkin, radicchio, radish, red cabbage, rocket, spinach, swede, sweet potato, Swiss chard, tomato, turnip, watercress, yam.

Fruit:

Apple, apricot, banana, blackberries, blackcurrants, blueberries, cherries, cranberries, damson, dates, dragon fruit, durian, elderberries, fig, gooseberry, grape, grapefruit, guava, jackfruit, kiwi, kumquat, lemon, lime, lychee, mango, melon, mulberries, nectarine, orange, papaya, passionfruit, peach, pear, persimmon, pineapple, plum, pomegranate, quince, raspberries, redcurrants, rhubarb, satsuma, starfruit, strawberries, tamarind, tangerine, ugli fruit, watermelon, yuzu.

Extra challenge 1: Start to cut back on sugar. This doesn't just mean jam or desserts. If you regularly have fruit juice or fruit-based smoothies, you'd be better off cutting these out altogether and eating whole fruit instead. The blitzing process all but destroys all the fibre so the fruits end up being little more than liquid sugar.

Extra challenge 2: If you drink alcohol every day, try three days (it doesn't matter which ones) with no alcohol.

Lunch on the go or at work

It's still not easy to find high-fibre options when you are out but here are four I like:

From M&S:
Roasted Butternut & Goat's Cheese Salad with giant couscous, lentils and balsamic dressing has **9.4g fibre**.
Super Nutty Wholefood (quinoa, edamame bean, soybean, almonds, peanuts and pistachios with soy and ginger dressing) also has **9.4g fibre**.

From Pret:
Hummus and Falafel Mezze Salad has **11.8g fibre**.
Avo and Herb Wrap has 6.7g, and could be followed with **Dark Chocolate Salted Almonds (3.5g fibre)** to enable you to just scrape over the 10g mark.

Fab fibre tip 4

You can increase your fibre by taking a fibre supplement. But you will be missing out on all the additional health benefits that come from eating it naturally, such as vitamins, minerals and antioxidants.

ANTIOXIDANTS RULE OK

You may remember that earlier I talked about how good antioxidants are for us, and ways to get more of them into our diet. Vegetables, fruit, herbs and spices are the best sources. A good rule of thumb is that the more deeply coloured the fruit or vegetable, and the less likely it is to go brown after being cut open, the more antioxidants it contains. So vegetables with high levels include broccoli, spring greens and tomatoes, while lemons, oranges, mangoes and cherries trump apples and bananas. But the top values go to herbs and spices. A single teaspoon of dried oregano, for example, can double your meal's antioxidants.

According to Dr Michael Greger, antioxidant-rich foods can be particularly beneficial if you are at risk of a stroke.

A study of 30,000 women over 12 years by Swedish researchers

Fabulous fibre snack options

As your primary goal is to eat 10-12 per cent fewer calories, it's a good idea to limit your snacks as much as possible. But if you're in danger of cracking – eat crackers! Preferably water biscuits or fine-milled oatcakes, as they are low in fat and sugar – with some cheese (cottage cheese is ideal; failing that, choose a hard cheese like Gruyere or Manchego rather than a fattier one like Brie).

Other options:
1 slice multigrain bread with half a tablespoon peanut butter
Apple or pear with a stick of hard cheese
Small serving of hummus with carrot and pepper sticks

found those who ate the most antioxidant-rich diet had the lowest stroke risk.[18] There was a similar finding in a study of both men and women in Italy.

What these diets do, says Dr Greger, is to prevent the circulation of oxidised fats in the bloodstream that can damage small blood vessels in the brain. They can also help decrease artery stiffness, prevent blood clots from forming and lower blood pressure.

HOW TO KEEP TRE ON TRACK

The more you practise TRE, the easier it becomes. Remember, you're only aiming for the mildest form – a 12-hour fast each day in which you eat nothing after your evening meal until breakfast 12 hours later.

The trick is to identify before you start the things that are likely to knock you off course, so that you can prepare strategies to stop that happening. Think about what you could do differently in the evenings so that you occupy your brain in another way, which in turn will distract you from snacking thoughts.

The first thing to do is empty your kitchen cupboards of any fast, ultra-processed unhealthy snacks. If you share your home with anyone who *does* eat them, then at least shove them all into a bag and move them somewhere – preferably slightly inaccessible, for example, under the stairs, where they can still find them but you can fairly easily avoid them.

---

18 Total Antioxidant Capacity of Diet and Risk of Stroke. *Stroke: J. Amer. Heart Assoc.*, 2011 – www.ahajournals.org/doi/pdf/10.1161/STROKEAHA.111.635557

However, if you're an inveterate snacker, there's still the danger that after finishing your evening meal at around 7 or 7.30pm, you'll find yourself in the kitchen an hour or two later, halfway through whatever you're watching on Netflix, rustling up cheese and crackers or dates with walnuts. It doesn't matter that those are healthy, high-fibre snacks – if you have them now, you're breaking your fast and with it all the repair and renewal work in your body that it would otherwise be activating.

What to do? Here are a few suggestions:

- Instead of watching TV, play a game or call a friend. The craving for a snack is habitual, and so less likely to be triggered when you break out of your routine and do something different.
- Plan treats: have a luxurious bath, go for a manicure or pedicure if you have a nail bar or salon that opens late, or even book a massage.
- Go for a walk after you've eaten. It will flatten the glucose spike so that you won't want a snack.
- Get busy: you could always clean out that cupboard, drawer or room you've been meaning to sort for months but never got round to. The combination of physical activity and cognitive activation – deciding what to keep and how to reorganise – means your brain is much less likely to think about a snack. Plus, you'll feel extremely smug when it's done!
- Choose a book you really want to read or a podcast you know you'll enjoy and go to bed early. Assuming you don't routinely snack in bed, it's very unlikely you'll think about it while you're reading or listening – and when you've finished you can just drift off to sleep.
- Above all, keep reminding yourself why you're doing this: to avoid that dread slide into frailty, immobility and chronic

disease. To be able to move easily and vigorously well into your 80s, 90s and beyond; to be able to run for the bus, go for a long walk, enjoy going on holiday, see friends, have fun. To maintain your independence and your energy. To live a long and vibrantly healthy life. Is it really worth giving up all that for the sake of a measly mid-evening snack?

Fabulous fibre desserts

While I'm all for living as long as possible, life is too short to have no treats. It's just a question of rethinking them (although rules are made to be broken *occasionally*, so sometimes it's also good to have whatever takes your fancy!). Here are some ideas:

- Raspberries and strawberries with chopped hazelnuts, one large square dark chocolate, grated, and just a little cream...
- Apple crumble with oats and nuts rather than standard flour mix
- Flapjacks with high nut content
- Caramelised pears with ginger, cinnamon and crème fraîche or Greek yoghurt
- My go-to cake is an orange and almond cake – made with two whole oranges, including the rind, and ground almonds, as well as sugar and eggs. No idea how much fibre it contains but it has to be more than most cakes – and it's delicious. Serve with crème fraîche if you like, but it's very moist so can be eaten on its own. Yum. Here's a link to the recipe I use if you fancy trying it: www.recipetineats.com/flourless-orange-cake/#wprm-recipe-container-51724

LIFELINE: THE TINY MOVEMENT YOU CAN DO WHILE SITTING THAT REDUCES BLOOD SUGAR BY 50 PER CENT

Imagine if you could keep your blood sugar level down just by sitting. Sounds ridiculous, doesn't it? But thanks to a professor of exercise physiology at Houston University, it's actually entirely doable. And easy.

Not only will it lower the glucose in your blood (blood sugar) by as much as 50 per cent, but it will also lower your insulin response too – by more, in many cases, than if you lost up to 15 per cent of your weight or exercised fanatically – and keep it low for three hours or more after eating.

As if that weren't enough, it also lowers your 'bad' cholesterol – LDL triglycerides – and may even help you lose weight.

It's the discovery of Professor Marc Hamilton (the scientist who 20 years ago sounded the alarm about the terrible damage we do to our bodies by sitting down all day.) And it's achieved by doing what he calls soleus muscle push-ups, or SPUs, when you're sitting.

Our soleus muscles are in our calves and it's important to do the push-up correctly. Luckily, it's extremely easy to do – and the wonderful thing about it is if you're doing it right, you won't feel any muscle fatigue whatsoever.

All you have to do is have your feet on the ground, preferably with your toes underneath your knees, so that if you drew a line between them it would be more or less straight. And you can do it with your shoes on – no need to be barefoot.

Now, starting off with just one foot, push lightly down on the ball of your foot. As you do so, your heel should lift off the floor. That's because the soleus muscle in your calf has contracted, or shortened, bringing your heel up with it. Then bring your heel back down, and repeat.

And that's it. You get a better effect if you both feet at once, and it couldn't be easier. Even very unfit people can do this movement for HOURS – that's right, hours – without getting fatigued.

In his trial,[19] Professor Hamilton deliberately recruited people who were unfit and didn't enjoy exercise. They were able to do SPUs for 270 minutes – that's four and a half hours – without feeling muscle soreness or cramps or any discomfort. That's how long it took for a 50 per cent reduction in blood sugar – but it began decreasing after just 30 minutes.

Although the soleus muscle is just one of the 600 muscles in your body, making up just 1 per cent of your body mass, it burns an enormous amount of fuel for its size. More oxygen is burned by the soleus doing these contractions than by any other exercise, including running to exhaustion on a treadmill. And the reason this exercise is so good for controlling blood sugar is because when engaged like this, the soleus uses the glucose in our blood as its fuel.

Professor Hamilton is now doing more studies to look at the other benefits of doing SPUs. He suspects it will help improve longevity in other ways.

He aims to do SPUs for half the time he is sitting and estimates he does around 60,000 a day. Here are his tips for starting:

1. **The goal is to make it a sustainable habit.** Each and every day. Most find it feasible some of every hour of the day when doing normal seated behaviours you do anyway.

---

19 A potent physiological method to magnify and sustain soleus oxidative metabolism improves glucose and lipid regulation. *iScience*, 2022 – doi: 10.1016/j. isci.2022.104869

2. **Make a short-term goal for two days for a high frequency and brief duration that you know you can do with a strong commitment (such as 'I will do SPUs for 2–5 min 20 times today.')** The average person sits down more than 20 times a day for a total of 600 minutes. So there is plenty of opportunity if you commit.

3. **Then after that short-term victory, you are ready to make a one month commitment.** You choose how many times you do it each day. For me personally, I find it easiest to simply tell myself that I will spend at least half of all my sitting time doing SPUs, every hour I sit and every day. But I find that once I get going, there's no reason to stop! It makes me feel energised knowing I am constantly saturating my body with the effects of a healthy low stress kind of muscle metabolism.'

Brain food

The best foods for the brain are the same ones that protect your heart and your blood vessels, according to Harvard Medical School. These include green leafy vegetables, fatty fish such as salmon and cod, berries, walnuts (which research shows may improve memory) and coffee, which according to studies doesn't just give us a short-term boost but appears to also help solidify new memories.

COMMON EXCUSES/
PSYCHOLOGICAL GET-OUTS

You'll find no judgement here. Equally though (because I've done it myself), I know how easy it is to make excuses and to talk yourself out of eating better and exercising more. Recognise any of these?

- I really don't have the time to do this properly now – I'll start again when things are less busy.
- Nothing like this has ever worked for me before and this won't either, so there's no point carrying on with it and making myself miserable in the process.
- No one really cares whether I do it or not, so what's the point?
- My husband/wife/friend says they like me just as I am and to stop worrying.

Well, here's the point. YOU really do matter. This is YOUR life. No one else's. If you can't make time for looking after yourself, for caring about yourself, for helping the truly magnificent machine that is your body to become strong, healthy and resilient so you can live as long as possible as well as possible, who can?

And yes, maybe your partner or friend really does like you just the way you are. But maybe that's because they're worried that if you change, they'll be left behind. That if you get stronger, healthier, fitter, younger, you won't want to be with them any more. Or that you'll judge them and find them wanting.

Either way, if they are suggesting you don't try to improve your health, it means that actually they care more about themselves than about you.

Because someone who really cared about you would say, 'Yes, go for it! Get healthier, stronger, younger, fitter! That's fantastic news, because I love you and want the very best for you.'

GOLDEN RULES

- **Plan your snacks.** As Professor Kraus points out, to reduce your calories by the golden 10–12 per cent all you need to do is avoid the temptation of the Starbucks scone (or muffin, or lemon drizzle cake, or whatever...) And that's much easier to do when you've got a healthier lower-calorie snack readily to hand for when hunger strikes. Try half a walnut sandwiched between two halves of a date or a rye cracker with slivers of a hard cheese such as Manchego or Gruyere – quick, easy, satisfying and filling.
- **Plan a week's worth of menus and stick to them.** The simpler the better.
- **Be more tortoise!** Don't beat yourself up if one day you eat more than you planned. The odd lapse really doesn't matter. It's so easy to think, that's it, I knew I couldn't do it, and use that as an excuse to abandon the whole plan. See it for what it is – a lapse. No one is perfect and life has a habit of getting in the way of even the best-laid plans. The most important thing is to get back on it the next day.
- **Don't forget herbs and spices.** They make a huge difference to the flavour, and hence our enjoyment, of food. And they are high in antioxidants and flavones – plant compounds also found in vegetables and fruits that have an anti-inflammatory effect; the single most anti-inflammatory food is turmeric,

followed by ginger and garlic. And don't forget – they're included in the 30 different fruits and vegetables you're aiming to eat each week. Liven up broccoli with fresh or dried chillies, sesame seeds and a drizzle of olive oil; sex up spinach with lemon juice, a drizzle of olive oil and black pepper; add a generous handful of chopped oregano and basil to ratatouille, flat-leaf parsley to carrots and fresh dill to poached salmon; slather lemon zest and rosemary mixed with olive oil on chicken before cooking… the more you experiment, the more you'll find combinations you love.

- Buy lentils, chickpeas and any other beans/legumes that you like to store in your cupboard as replacements for pasta, potatoes and rice.
- Ditch any biscuits, sweets or cakes – if they're not in your home, you won't be tempted to eat them.
- Buy the nuts you enjoy – almonds, pistachios, pecans, walnuts: a variety is good.
- Remind yourself of your motivation: write down a few key words on post-it notes to remind yourself why you are doing this. Then stick them on your desk, in the kitchen, on the stairs and anywhere else you are likely to see them around your home or at work.
- Think of someone who inspires you and do it for them when the going gets tough.
- When you crave something to eat, get up and move.

* * *

Having experienced the benefits of eating more plants, I hope you'll be feeling so well and energised you'll want to continue.

You will be eating incredibly well, feeling full instead of hankering for something sweet, and probably losing a bit of weight to boot.

You should now have a rough log in your head of foods that are fibre-rich so that it is easy to adjust your choices. Your body may also lead the way in this, by actively craving some foods that previously you would hardly have considered. Before I started including beans and pulses in my diet I barely gave them a thought. Now I find myself craving them – especially butter beans.

The important thing to understand now is that by embarking on this three-week programme, you have begun to radically transform not just your health and longevity but also your psychological approach to the food your body needs. It is up to you what you do next. I urge you to adopt some of its strategies permanently.

Incidentally, you can do TRE as often as you like. But, even if you do it just three or four days out of every month, it will have a major impact on your longevity and health. You will find that, just as reducing your consumption of foods high in fat and sugar reduces your cravings, so eating less often will make you feel better and better until it becomes the way you *prefer* to eat.

The same, I'm glad to say, goes for exercise. The only way to do more exercise is to learn to love it – and in the next chapter I'm going to show you how.

Why an orange is much better for you than a glass of orange juice

When you drink a glass of orange juice, most of the fibre – the body of the orange – has been removed. So what you're drinking is a lot of sugar, with vitamin C. This results in a sugar spike – too much sugar flooding your body at once, which after the initial energy rush will in turn lead to a sugar dip, resulting in you feeling tired and headache-y. That will make you want more sugar, and a vicious cycle starts.

Fibre helps your body regulate sugar as it slows down digestion. If instead of juice you eat the whole orange, the fibre allows your body to process the absorption of sugar much more steadily.

Why coffee is good for you (and when to drink it)

Coffee really is good for you – and especially good for your heart. An impressive 76 studies of more than a million people in total show that coffee reduces the risk of death from heart disease by about a fifth.

There are some studies that suggest it may even help survival after a heart attack. Plus it reduces the risk of breast, colon and prostate cancer. The optimum is around three cups a day.

Coffee is a major source of plant polyphenols – self-defence chemicals created by plants to protect them against predators or severe weather. These polyphenols play a key role in controlling both chronic inflammation and blood sugar.

Just remember it's a good idea to have your last coffee somewhere between midday and 2pm, to avoid it disrupting your sleep. (For more on when to drink it, turn to p169).

3
MOVING MORE

Wait! Before you skip this chapter because you hate/are bored by/ are no good at/can't be bothered with exercise and would much rather flick forward to find out how to have better sleep, consider this amazing fact:

You only have to walk a mile every day (that's around 2000 steps) to reduce your chances of dying by almost a third – 30 per cent.

Interested? Good. Because I'm here to tell you not only why exercise can save your life, but how to fall in love with it as well.

So, here's how to start. It doesn't matter if you were rubbish at sport at school, always got picked last for the team, can't run to catch a bus... whatever. You can walk one mile. You do have to walk briskly. It can't be an indolent stroll. But it is only for 20 minutes.

Just try it – right now, if possible. If you have a phone, chances are it can measure a mile for you in maps, and/or it can measure your steps. But either way it doesn't matter. All you have to do is walk briskly for 20 minutes, enough to get slightly out of breath but not so much that you can't talk.

And... that's it.

When you finish, you'll realise you feel better than when you started. Your mood will have lifted, because exercise gives you a dopamine hit (the same hit people get from taking drugs) and that's why if you do it often enough, it becomes addictive. The difference being that exercise is good for every single part of your body, including your brain, and considerably reduces your chances of getting every major disease, including dementia.

You don't have to be sporty or athletic or young or thin to do the exercises in this chapter. Anyone can do them – and everyone will feel better afterwards. That's the power of exercise. And that's how you can start to learn to love it (more on which later).

* * *

'When it comes to exercise, what everyone wants to know,' explains Professor Bill Kraus, 'is, "how little can I do?"' It was Professor Kraus, a cardiologist at Duke University in North Carolina, who – as you may remember from the last chapter – was involved from the beginning in the CALERIE research study. This was the two-year trial that set out to discover the impact of cutting calorie intake by 25 per cent a day.

So he has come up with the answer to the 'How little can I do?' question. It was his research paper that showed that 2000 steps a day is all you need to do to reduce your chances of dying by almost a third. It's also all you need to do to achieve the 150 minutes of moderate-intensity exercise that's recommended in both the US and the UK national guidelines. 'Here's the math,' he explains. 'Moderate-intensity activity is about 3 miles an hour. Every mile is around 2000 steps. So if we are telling people to do 150 minutes, which is two and a half hours, of moderate intensity physical activity a week at 3 miles an hour that calculates out to 7 miles a week or around 14–15,000 steps a week, or around 2000 steps a day.

'On top of that I'm going to give you 5000 steps a day. That's what you get from what we call activities of daily living – ADL. Things like going from the bedroom to the bathroom, the kitchen to the front door, going up and downstairs, walking to the store for some groceries. That calculates out to 7000 steps a day. And it turns out that 7000 steps a day is all you need, not 10,000.

'But the point is this: you have to be intentional about the activities of daily living. Take the stairs. Walk when you can. If you go to Starbucks, just to get a coffee, don't go to the drive thru. Park the car and walk in.

'Because what our research shows is that it doesn't matter how you accumulate the physical activity. It doesn't have to be in minimum-length bouts. Every minute counts.'

A recent meta-analysis[1] of studies published in the *European Journal of Preventive Cardiology* proved this point. It included more than 17 cohort studies with a total of more than 225,000 adults, average age 64, from multiple countries. They were tracked on average for seven years. The researchers concluded the following: each increase of 1000 steps you do a day decreases your risk of premature death by 15 per cent.

And even more definitive proof, as if it were needed, of the benefits of exercise came in another recent study by Professor Kraus's wife, Professor Virginia Kraus, also at Duke (they are a powerhouse couple – he a cardiologist, she a rheumatologist, with seven professorships between them and umpteen published papers).

---

1 The association between daily step count and all-cause and cardiovascular mortality: a meta-analysis, *Eur. J. Prev. Card.*, 2023 – doi:10.1093/eurjpc/zwad229

Professor Virginia Kraus has used a revolutionary new form of data analysis to discover direct causes of longevity from medically accessible data. The analysis considers nearly 200 variables and their millions of combinations to uncover the underlying direct causes of longevity in older adults, and the results are startling. The research, on data from 1500 people aged 71 and over, found that the two most important determinants of longevity in older adults are physical activity and a component of HDL or 'good' cholesterol known as small HDL particles. The density of these particles matters far more than your levels of 'bad' LDL cholesterol.

Not only that but the research also shows that having had heart attacks, strokes, cancer, diabetes or high blood pressure did not play the most important role in predicting people's longevity. Exercise, small HDL particles and not smoking mattered much more.

I ask her what her longevity advice would be to someone in their 50s or 60s who doesn't exercise. 'I would say, get a smart watch, and do 8000 steps a day,' she replies firmly. 'The mortality curve drops precipitously with the littlest bit of exercise, the littlest bit of activities of daily living.'

She recommends 8000 steps a day even for those with osteoarthritis – which as a rheumatologist is her special area of interest (for more on osteoarthritis, see box on p101).

* * *

When I tell Steve Harridge, professor of human and applied physiology at King's College London and co-director of Ageing Research at King's (ARK), that my biological age is 20, he says immediately: 'So you do a lot of exercise?'

The way he views it, people who exercise should be the benchmark for studying human ageing. They are the ones who are ageing as they should – it's people who DON'T exercise who are deviating from what our bodies were intended to do and therefore from the healthy lifespan we should all be enjoying.

In other words, it's not that the exercisers are making themselves younger. It's that those who don't exercise are making themselves older than they need to be.

'You're not reversing ageing by exercising regularly, you're accelerating your decline by not exercising regularly,' he says. 'It's a complete philosophical switch.'

Professor Harridge is part of a group of top academics around the world who published a consensus report on international guidelines for exercise recommendations for older adults.[2] The report concluded that insufficient exercise is a 'potent risk factor' for all cause and cardiovascular mortality, together with obesity, muscle loss, frailty, stroke, heart disease, diabetes and cancer, and that exercise (defined as structured physical activity) helps prevent all these, and should be prescribed as a medicine.

He believes that exercise is even more important than what we eat.

'That's not to say nutrition is not important – it is, very – but I think exercise tends to get put into a second division of importance, when it should be at the top.

'I don't disagree at all with promoting optimal nutrition. It's just that many people spend so much time angsting about what they should be eating, believing that a healthy diet alone is sufficient for health when it's not. So, a little less time angsting about food and more time being physically active would be a better approach. Exercise is fundamental to health and to ageing well.

---

2 International Exercise Recommendations In Older Adults. *J. Nutr. Health & Aging*, 2021 – pubmed.ncbi.nlm.nih.gov/34409961/

'The whole package of exercise and nutrition comes together as a lifestyle choice. Being physically active, eating a well-balanced mixed diet, maintains overall fitness and helps maintain an appropriate body weight. This is in addition to other factors such as sleeping well, not smoking and drinking alcohol in moderation, which all contribute to one's health. Smoking is a definite no-no, and the rise in vaping is very worrying and a potential disaster in the making.

'While drinking no alcohol would be ideal, for many it is an enjoyable part of life and the guideline of 14 units per week seems a sensible one. Having aspects of life that are enjoyable is essential, and these include having a good social connection and family network.'

Even when leading your best life, he points out, 'there is no *guarantee* of living longer and healthier. But we do at least have the power to move the odds in our favour, by making the right lifestyle choices.'

So what should we do for the best chance of ageing well? 'It's important to differentiate lifespan from healthspan. While modern medicine is able to keep us alive for longer than before, these extra years of life are for many not healthy ones. Being physically active and exercising reduces the risk of getting cardiovascular disease, becoming obese and developing metabolic diseases like type 2 diabetes. Ideally, we want to live healthily for as long as we can and reduce as much as possible the period towards the end of life where we are in poor health and potentially reliant on lots of medication and the care of others. In other words, we want to compress our morbidity.

'While plenty of diseases are not related to lifestyle, by living healthily you can reduce the risk of those that are. And for many, that may simply mean moving more.

'Dame Sally Davies, the former chief medical officer, once said that "if physical activity were a drug, we'd talk about it as a miracle cure", because it does so many good things to the body. That's why it's so difficult to replicate in the form of medication. As well as your heart and muscles, you're training the immune system, the brain, the central nervous system, all of which contribute to your integrative physiology. Pharmaceuticals, on the other hand, tend to target very specific things. But we can also view exercise as medicine, with different types of exercise being like different drugs targeting different things, depending on the types of exercise you do. For many people who are inactive, just moving around more, for example, walking to the shops rather than driving, can be really beneficial.

'But the reality is that it's extremely difficult to get people to change behaviour and be more active, and vast swathes of the population do way less than the recommended levels.

'Our bodies evolved to suit the needs of being hunter-gatherers. So we are biologically designed to be more active and similarly we are also designed to go for periods without eating – namely, fasting. Both exercise and periods of fasting are types of stressors, but they are good stressors that benefit the body, which responds and adapts accordingly.'

Hate exercise? Then consider this.

- Every year after the age of 60, you may lose about 1 per cent of muscle mass, 1 per cent of leg strength and 3–4 per cent of leg power. So by the time you are 80 you may have lost 20 per cent of your muscle mass, and between 20 and 80 per cent of your muscle function.

'This is driven by both ageing and inactivity,' says Professor Harridge. 'Resistance exercise is the most effective way of maintaining mass and function as we age. Not by affecting ageing, but by tackling the inactive part. We know from studying older master athletes who train incredibly hard that they still decline in performance as they age. But in these individuals this decline is driven by "ageing" and not inactivity accompanying ageing.'

So what sort of exercise should you be doing? The answer is the one you enjoy, as that's the one you'll be most likely to do consistently. But ideally it should combine both resistance and cardio exercise, as our bodies need both to function at their best.

WHAT IS CARDIO EXERCISE?

Cardio exercise is any activity that gets your heart rate up and increases blood flow – for example, running, brisk walking uphill, rowing, skipping.

Doing vigorous exercise of this kind – enough to get your breathing to the point that you can still just about talk but can't hold a long conversation with proper sentences – causes your muscles to use more blood and oxygen, which in turn means your heart and lungs have to work harder. The more cardio you do, the stronger your heart and lungs will get. Not only that, but oxygenated blood then pumps through your entire body, including your brain, providing extraordinary benefits.

The increased blood flow to the brain helps the production of molecules that stimulate neurons to grow in the brain for maintenance and function.

Cardio exercise also raises 'good' cholesterol (HDL) and lowers 'bad' cholesterol (LDL) and triglycerides, the fats that circulate through your body when you eat more calories than you expend (typically from a diet high in saturated fat and sugar – foods like burgers, biscuits and cake).

Cardio helps keep your blood pressure low, and your arteries clear, by forcing more blood to flow more quickly through the arteries. This in turn helps your blood vessels remodel and stay healthy.

As if all that weren't enough, exercise also promotes the growth of mitochondria – these are the energy factories of each cell, which use oxygen to burn fat and carbohydrates – improving the body's ability to use sugar and reduce inflammation.

VO2MAX AND WHY IT MATTERS

Most experts, including Professor Harridge and Peter Attia, a medical doctor and expert on longevity, agree that the gold-standard measure of health and physical fitness is VO2max – that is, the maximum rate at which the body can use oxygen. In fact, if you have below-average VO2max for your age and sex, you are at greater risk of dying than if you smoke.[3]

---

3 As Peter Attia points out in his excellent book *Outlive*: 'A 2018 study in the *Journal of the American Medical Association* that followed more than 120,000 people found that higher VO2max was associated with lower mortality across the board. The fittest people had the lowest mortality rates by a big margin. A person who smokes has a 40 per cent greater risk of all-cause mortality (ie, risk of dying at any moment), than someone who does not smoke. But someone with below-average VO2max for their age and sex is at double the risk of all-cause mortality compared to someone in the top quarter. So poor cardiorespiratory fitness carries a greater relative risk of death than smoking. And someone in the bottom quarter for their age and sex is four times more like to die than someone in the top quarter. These results were confirmed by a much larger and more recent study, published in 2022 in the *Journal of the American College of Cardiology*. Data from US veterans aged

And at any given age, says Professor Harridge, VO2max is higher in those who exercise. 'In practical terms, this equates to a "buying back" of years of function compared with sedentary people,' he says, and adds that, while many believe that mitochondrial dysfunction and lowering of the body's sensitivity to insulin are inevitable consequences of ageing, studies show that both mitochondrial function and overall metabolic health are substantially better in people who exercise, irrespective of age. And the good news, says Professor Harridge, is that even if you've never exercised, once you start, these levels can be improved.

WHAT IS RESISTANCE EXERCISE?

Any weight-bearing exercise, for example lifting weights, doing push-ups or pull-ups, stresses the fibres in your muscles, which forces them to become stronger. It also helps prevent bone loss, and improves cholesterol levels as well as your muscles' ability to use sugar.

Like cardio, resistance exercise also benefits the brain: one consequence is that your brain learns the patterns of movement that allow you to balance better more quickly and adapt to heavy loads.

So resistance exercise, done regularly, not only prevents the body from getting frail, but also enables you to respond much better to a sudden event, such as tripping on something, without losing your footing.

30–95, men and women, found a nearly identical result: someone in the least fit 20 per cent has a four times greater risk of dying than someone in the top 2 per cent. "Being unfit carried a greater risk than any of the cardiac risk factors examined," the authors concluded.'

Muscle loss, or sarcopenia, which is when it reaches a level where it is defined as a disease – like osteoporosis bone loss – is the reason so many older people have saggy bottoms, flabby thighs and dangly 'bingo wings'. Not a great look – and not an inevitable one.

But even if you don't care about how you look, you should care about how you function. Because those cottonwool thighs and that sinking bottom mean that when you stumble or trip, it will be that much harder to keep your balance. When you climb stairs or walk fast, you'll have to stop, not just because your lungs are burning but because your legs are too weak to continue. Your arms won't be strong enough to lift a small grandchild.

Dr Attia (whose celebrity fans include Hugh Jackman and Gwyneth Paltrow, to name but two) urges everyone to start thinking now about what they would still like to be able to do when they are 90. The options he suggests we consider include being able to open a jar, walk fast uphill for a mile and a half, climb four flights of stairs in three minutes, and (look away now, children) still have sex.

Most people, when asked, he says, reply that they would like to be still able to do all those things when they are 90. In which case, they need to begin resistance training and cardio exercise right now, so that they have as long as possible to build and maintain strength and power before they reach their eighth or ninth decade.

Once you're over 65, explains Dr Attia, breaking a hip can mean death: 'There's a 15 to 30 per cent chance of death in the next 12 months, and of those who don't die, 50 per cent will never regain full function. It's an awful statistic.'

He passionately believes that when it comes to extending your life healthily, exercise is the most important factor.

If you've always hated exercise and think there's no point starting now, I urge you to think again.

CAN EXERCISE HELP WARD OFF DISEASE?

The answer is an emphatic yes. Professor Bill Kraus believes one significant reason for this is that exercise promotes autophagy – the clearing out of toxins from cells. Research by him and others at Duke using the relatively new science of metabolomics (large-scale studies of small molecules) is beginning to point to what may be the earliest markers of cardiac disease, but they still do not know what causes the molecules to behave in the way that creates those markers. That work is ongoing.

Professor Kraus is clear, however, that anything that can increase autophagy is beneficial: 'And I know that in muscle, exercise activates autophagy.'

HOW EXERCISE CAN
REJUVENATE YOUR HEART

Dr Benjamin Levine is a renowned sports cardiologist at the University of Texas Southwestern Medical Center who has long been fascinated by how exercise improves health in general and the heart in particular.

He has discovered that even in late middle age, if you exercise in the right way, you can actually make your heart younger.

The heart, he explains, starts to shrink in late middle age – which might be younger than you think; he defines middle age as starting at age 50 (and ending at 65).

And if you're younger than that, don't be too complacent – Dr Levine adds that the heart starts to stiffen in what he calls early middle age, that is from age 35 to 49.

His study,[4] a randomised controlled trial, took two years and involved a group of 53 men and women aged between 45 and 64, with an average height of 169cm and average weight of 75kg.

Crucially, they were all sedentary, defined for the purposes of the study as people who did not exercise consistently – and if they did ever exercise, did so for less than 30 minutes fewer than three times a week. They had no specific heart or circulatory problems or disease.

They were divided into two groups. One, the control group, did a combination of yoga, balance and strength training three times a week. The other group – the exercise training group – were progressively worked harder and harder with cardio exercise, so that after six months they were training 5–6 hours a week.

From months 6 to 10, their weekly training consisted of two high-intensity sessions, where they did four repetitions of exercising flat out at 95 per cent of their maximum capacity for four minutes, each followed by three minutes' recovery (known as 4×4 interval training); one long endurance session of at least an hour, and one 30-minute base pace session. These were supplemented by strength training sessions twice a week.

After 10 months, the 4×4 sessions were cut down to just one a week and the training continued for another year. The results were astonishing: in the exercise training group their hearts actually got bigger and their arteries more elastic.

Their hearts processed oxygen more efficiently and were notably less stiff; the hearts of the control group didn't change.

A key part of the exercise regimen was the interval training, which was based on an old Norwegian ski team workout. Dr

---

4 Reversing the Cardiac Effects of Sedentary Aging in Middle Age. *Circulation*, 2018 – www.ahajournals.org/doi/full/10.1161/CIRCULATIONAHA.117.030617

It's never too late

Sceptics or professional exercise loathers may like to consider the astonishing achievements of Richard Morgan, a former baker who lives in Ireland and at the age of 94 is a four-time champion indoor rower, winning his last title in 2022.

But here's the truly mind-blowing fact: **he didn't start rowing until he was 73 – and before that had done no structured training or exercise at all.**

So how did he do it? According to a study published in the *Journal of Applied Physiology* in November 2023,[1] he achieved this by being consistent in both his training (indoor rowing every day and resistance training two or three times a week) and his diet (high in protein, with very little alcohol).

He trained on a rowing machine for 40 minutes a day, covering 30 kilometres a week. But most of this rowing training – 70 per cent – was at what is called zone 2 intensity, where your perceived effort is around 5 or 6 out of 10; of the remaining training, 20 per cent was at a higher intensity of 7–8, and 10 per cent at maximal effort. His resistance training two or three times a week consisted of three sets of lunges, rows and curls with weights, taken close to, or to, failure.

Exceptionally, his body composition showed extremely high muscle mass, at 80 per cent. And his peak heart rate – 153 beats per minute – is the highest ever recorded for someone in their 90s. (Bear in mind that by then he had been training for 20 years – so not something to just rush in and try for yourself at home!)

---

1 Physiological characteristics of a 92-yr-old four-time world champion indoor rower. *J. Applied Phys.*, 2023 – doi:10.1152/japplphysiol.00698.2023

His grandson Lorcan Daly, an assistant lecturer in exercise science at the Technological University of the Shannon in Ireland, and one of the authors of the study, says the findings are unique: 'They tell us that fitness is very responsive. You can start at any time. It's never too late.'

As Professor Lieberman points out, in hunter-gatherer tribes, such as the Hadza in Tanzania, elderly grandparents are often more active than younger parents. The body's mechanisms that allow us to do weight-bearing activities remain effective as we age, if only we would use them.

Levine says that by pushing as hard as possible for four minutes, the heart is stressed and forced to function more efficiently. Repeating the intervals makes both it and the circulatory system stronger.

However, after a certain age, he found – around 70 – the heart can't be changed in the same way. This doesn't mean you shouldn't start exercising at the age of 70, he says – you will still reduce your risk of sudden cardiac death, you will improve the endothelial lining of the arteries so that the blood flow is more efficient, and you will at the very least preserve your aerobic capacity.

HOW EXERCISE PROTECTS AGAINST CANCER

The rates of many cancers are rising: for example, breast cancer rates in Britain doubled in the 83 years between 1921 and 2004.

Numerous studies have examined the relationship between physical activity and cancer and all show that those who exercise regularly and moderately are at substantially lower risk.

As Professor Daniel Lieberman, an evolutionary biologist at Harvard, explains in his excellent book *Exercised*, one analysis of six studies found that of 650,000 elderly people studied over 10 years, a quarter – one in four – died from cancer. But when the researchers delved deeper, they found that those who exercised at least moderately, or more, had between 25 and 30 per cent lower cancer rates.

'According to one estimate, three to four hours of moderate exercise a week is likely to reduce a woman's risk of breast cancer by 30 to 40 per cent, and both men and women's risk of colon cancer by 40 to 50 per cent,' says Professor Lieberman.

In other words, by doing regular, moderate exercise you can cut your risk of colon cancer by half.

HOW EXERCISE HELPS OSTEOARTHRITIS

There are two main causes of osteoarthritis, says Dr Virginia Kraus. The first is inflammation, and the second is chronic overuse. A third factor to consider is that genetically, some people are better able to regenerate their joints, and some people are also genetically more prone to inflammation. People in this last category have a hyper-reactivity to something called lipopolysaccharide, a product of the gut microbiome – and which, it turns out, is cleared by small particles in 'good' cholesterol, HDL.

Whatever the cause, though, exercise is crucial for both prevention and recovery. Professor Kraus recommends 8000 steps a day, which seems, she says, to be well tolerated even by people with knee or hip arthritis.

If walking on land is too painful, she recommends walking in the swimming pool, 'which is even better than being on the moon – on the moon the gravity is $\frac{1}{6}$ but in water is $\frac{1}{8}$ what it is on land, so you can get freedom of motion. And that's really really important for joint health,' she adds, 'because the cartilage in your joints doesn't have any blood supply. So the only way they get nutrition is through dynamic motion.'

GET A GRIP

A surprising indicator of overall health – and of how well we're ageing – is grip strength.[5] This is a classic example of use it or lose it, as it declines fairly rapidly with age – and we've all seen someone older struggle to get the lid off a jar. One study[6] in 2015 showed that loss of grip strength is an even more powerful predictor of death from cardiovascular disease than blood pressure.

You might be surprised to find how little grip strength you actually have, but it can be improved. Start by squeezing something squishy (like a stress ball), move on to weightlifting exercises such as deadlifts and farmer's carry (where you walk, without swinging your arms, carrying as heavy a weight as you can manage in each hand) and – simple but effective – seeing how long you can hang by your hands from a bar. If you want to measure your grip strength against the recommended levels for your age, you can even buy a hand grip strengthener – mine was around £30 on Amazon.

---

5 Grip Strength: An Indispensable Biomarker For Older Adults. *Clin. Interv. Aging*, 2019 –pmc.ncbi.nlm.nih.gov/articles/PMC6778477/#CIT0089
6 Prognostic value of grip strength. *Lancet*, 2018 – doi: 10.1016/ S0140-6736(14)62000-6. Epub 2015 May 13.

Dr Benjamin Levine's prescription for life

Dr Levine believes that exercise is medicine. This is his 'prescription for life', a weekly exercise plan for the average person who wants to be fit and healthy, which he believes people should do 'as part of their personal hygiene – just like brushing your teeth and taking a shower'. Importantly, you need to be exercising 4–5 times a week; 2–3 times isn't enough.

1 high-intensity workout of 30 minutes.
He favours the 4×4 routine mentioned above – four repetitions of exercising for four minutes at 95 per cent of your maximum intensity, each repetition followed by three minutes' recovery.

2 moderate-intensity sessions of at least 30 minutes.
You should be exercising hard enough to get a little bit of sweat on your brow, but still be able to talk (although not able to sing).

1 session of moderate-intensity aerobic activity for at least 1 hour.
It doesn't have to be running or swimming – it could be dancing or hiking or biking. The most important thing is that it is fun, something you enjoy.

1–2 sessions of strength training.
This could be weights at the gym but could also be strength yoga (as opposed to basic yoga) or Pilates.

BRAIN POWER: HOW EXERCISE IMPROVES YOUR MEMORY

Exercise is incredibly good for our brains too. In fact, it is probably the single best thing you can do to keep your brain healthy. And again, you don't need to do huge amounts to get the benefit. A 2023 study[7] co-authored by Dr David Merrill, director of the Pacific Brain Health Center at the Pacific Neuroscience Institute in Santa Monica, found that fewer than 4000 steps a day has a significant effect on memory.

The study looked at MRI brain scans from more than 10,100 people and found that those who regularly exercised had larger areas of both grey matter, which helps in processing information, and white matter, which connects different brain regions; and also a larger hippocampus, one of the main memory centres.

In 1999 a scientist called Henriette van Praag discovered that exercise actually causes the brain to grow new cells in the hippocampus. Six years later she showed in another paper[8] that even in old mice, running improved their memory and reversed the decline in their creation of brain cells by 50 per cent.

And, good news for anyone who has trouble sleeping: one recent study by the University of Portsmouth[9] demonstrated that in people who are sleep-deprived, 20 minutes of moderate exercise was even more beneficial for clearing out brain toxins than sleep.

---

7 Exercise-Related Physical Activity Relates to Brain Volumes in 10,125 Individuals. *J. Alz. Disease*, 2023– /dx.doi.org/ 10.3233/JAD-230740.
8 Exercise Enhances Learning and Hippocampal Neurogenesis in Aged Mice. *J. Neuroscience*, 2005 – doi: 10.1523/JNEUROSCI.1731-05.2005
9 The effects of sleep deprivation, acute hypoxia, and exercise on cognitive performance, *Phys. & Behav.*, 2024 – www.sciencedirect.com/science/article/pii/S0031938423003347?via%3Dihub

It's also been found that exercise, in particular high-intensity exercise, can help improve memory function. In 2010, researchers took a group of women aged between 55 and 85 with mild cognitive impairment – that is, they were starting to forget things, or repeat themselves – and asked them to do 45–60 minutes of high-intensity cardio exercise (at 75–85 per cent of their maximum heart rate) four times a week.

The control group did stretches for 45–60 minutes a day, four days a week, at 50 per cent or less of their maximum heart rate. After six months, scientists found that there was no difference in the memory function of the group who did the stretches, while that of the group who had done the aerobic exercise had improved.

Other studies using MRI scans show that aerobic exercise can actually reverse age-related shrinkage in the brain's memory centres, as well as improve blood flow in the brain and help preserve brain tissue.

Dr Flaminia Ronca, associate professor at UCL and the Institute of Sport, Exercise and Health, has a particular interest in how exercise affects the brain. Her research[10] is heartening: just 15 minutes of exercise, at an effort of 4 out of 10 – equivalent to brisk walking and broadly taken to mean that if you had to, you could still carry out a conversation for the duration – is enough to significantly increase brain activity in the prefrontal cortex. That's the part of the brain we use to think, pay attention, plan, make decisions and remember where we put our keys.

---

10 Decreased Exercise-Induced Changes in Prefrontal Cortex Hemodynamics Are Associated With Depressive Symptoms. *Front. Neuroergonomics*, 2022 – www.frontiersin.org/journals/neuroergonomics/articles/10.3389/fnrgo.2022.806485/full and
Body fat is predictive of acute effects of exercise on prefrontal hemodynamics and speed. *Neuropsychologia* – in press

Both high- and low-intensity exercise increase brain activity in the prefrontal cortex compared to resting, but higher intensities produce a stronger effect.

Dr Ronca says: 'We compared a light 15-minute cycle at an effort of 4 out of 10 to a 15-minute all-out maximal exercise test to exhaustion – they both increased brain activity, but the higher intensity promoted a significantly greater increase. The bigger picture is actually a bit more complicated than that, where moderate/vigorous intensities, such as jogging, tend to provide the greatest benefit compared to very light or very intense sessions."

In her study, those who were leaner and fitter showed a greater increase in brain activity.

'It seems that, while everyone benefits from a bit of exercise, people who are fitter and thinner might get a bigger "brain boost". To us this is very interesting, and we're still trying to find an explanation for it. It seems to be a cause-effect cycle. When we get fitter, our metabolism and brain systems seem to adapt in such a way that the body responds better to a bout of exercise, and therefore is able to draw a bigger benefit. For example, our studies suggest that while all participants show an improvement in brain activity during executive function tasks after 15 minutes' exercise, carrying more body fat reduced this effect. This might be linked to metabolic functions that can be affected by excess body fat and poor cardiovascular fitness. Other studies show that we respond better to endocannabinoids [neurotransmitters in the body that send signals between nerve cells] when we become fitter, which might explain why fitter people can get a significantly bigger mood boost from very strenuous aerobic exercise. So, everyone seems to benefit from a bit of jumping around, and the fitter we get, the more our brains learn to draw benefit from physical activity.'

COGNITIVE NEUROMOTOR EXERCISE

Along with cardio and resistance exercise there is a third form of workout we should all be doing: neuromotor exercise.

Neuromotor exercise is anything that requires you to move while also having to think, and it's extremely good for our brains. Yoga, Pilates and tai chi come under this umbrella, as do racquet sports – tennis, padel, pickleball, badminton, squash – and martial arts. Dance is also neuromotor exercise, and according to a recent study the one that works your brain the most. (If you doubt this, try going to dance classes to learn a complicated series of steps and see how well you get on…)

The great thing about all these activities is that they are fun. Racquet sports and dance also count as cardio exercise if you are really moving; but if you are doing yoga, Pilates or tai chi, or are the kind of tennis player who plays doubles and doesn't move around the court much, then you probably need to do some dedicated cardio too.

DUAL-TASKING BRAIN TRAINING:
THE NEXT BIG THING

Within neuromotor exercise is a category that is in its infancy at the moment but is probably the best thing you can possibly do for your brain health, and that is exercise combined not just with thinking – as in tennis or dancing – but with actual cognitive training.

In 2017, a UCLA post-doctoral neuroscientist, Sarah McEwen, had what she calls 'a hare-brained idea'. What would happen to the brain, she wondered, if you combined exercise and cognitive training, and did them at the same time? In other words – dual tasking.

She and a colleague – David Merrill, who is both a psychiatrist and neuroscientist – did a study[11] to investigate her theory, and they discovered that her idea wasn't so hare-brained. In fact, it was a breakthrough.

For the study they divided 55 participants aged between 60 and 75 years, all of whom had subjective memory loss, into two groups. For four weeks, twice a week, one group did memory games and drills while pedalling on a stationary bike. The other group also did memory games and drills, but only *after* they had done the stationary cycling. At the end of the four weeks, the group doing the simultaneous training showed significant improvements in verbal memory and complex attention ability.

Exercise with cognitive training is being pioneered in California, where I spent some time trying it out for myself and talking to some of the scientists at the forefront of developing it.

At the Pacific Brain Health Center – part of the Pacific Neuroscience Institute in Santa Monica, which among other incredible facilities has a special FitBrain gym – I talked to David Merrill about why this particular combination of cardio and cognitive exercise is so good for the brain.

The hippocampus is one of the only parts of the brain that can regenerate, he explains. This requires exercise. 'If you don't exercise, your muscles atrophy and your bones thin out. And the

---

11 Simultaneous Aerobic Exercise and Memory Training Program in Older Adults with Subjective Memory Impairments. *J. Alz. Disease*, 2018 – pmc.ncbi.nlm.nih. gov/articles/PMC5870016/

same thing happens in your brain's memory centre. Your brain shrinks down and it thins out.

'So when you do the opposite, it sends signals, which are also called trophic factors, from the muscles to the brain, and then the brain itself sends signals, brain-derived neurotrophic factors, to stay alive and then also to grow.

'So you can actually grow brain in the memory centres, and exercise supercharges it. It's a natural way of helping your brain grow. There's been decades of work showing that environmental enrichment, physical activity, exercise, cause the new brain cells that are born to sprout and connect to other things.

'What we do here in the brain gym, moving the body while challenging the brain, causes your brain cells to connect and stay connected, as well as causing the birth and connection of new cells. The old adage – use it or lose it – is really true. It's as true for the brain as it is for muscles.'

In the brain gym, I find myself confronted with various large machines. The first requires me to keep both feet together on a square in the centre of the floor. There are grab rails either side of me in case I lose my balance. In front of me is a large screen with four large dots – top, bottom and each side. As each one turns red, I have to keep one foot on the centre square and move the other to squares in front, behind or to the side, depending on which dot has turned red. My score, says the Pacific Brain Health Center's FitBrain director Ryan Glatt, is very good – which I find surprising, as doing it was far from easy.

Things are about to get worse, though.

We move on to the next machine. This has a large screen with four red target dots arranged in the same order as before – top, bottom, left and right. But this time a little black ball starts moving and now I have to not only move my foot and tap the relevant square on the floorpad, but time it so that it coincides with the exact moment the black ball hits the centre of the red target.

Just as I'm getting the hang of that, two other balls appear so that there are three moving randomly across the screen, in different directions towards different targets. I've got to work out where each one is going and when it's going to hit the centre of the target, while also moving one or other of my feet to press the appropriate square on the floorpad.

In a matter of seconds it's all chaos – I go forwards when I should be going backwards, and left instead of right. This is a LOT harder to do.

From there, we move on to two other machines and two more exercises. Again, they look quite straightforward – until you start doing them. It's taken less than 15 minutes for me to learn that this business of moving while at the same time trying to think is actually really difficult.

Which is why it is so effective. As Ryan reminds me, while doing them I am not only improving my brain function and memory; I'm also improving my balance. Remember Dr Peter Attia's warning that breaking a hip is a major cause of death in the over-65s? The most common way to break a hip is through a fall.

Ryan is 32 and fit – but, as he points out, if he's walking while also looking at his phone he can still twist his ankle. 'People don't fall when they're focused; they fall when they're distracted.'

I predict it won't be many years before brain gyms are commonplace. The smart thing would be for existing gyms to incorporate these machines and teach classes so that everyone, not just those lucky enough to live in California, can benefit from them.

Test how well you dual task

Try this simple test to see how well you dual task:

1. Walk across the room and ask someone to time you.
2. Now ask them to time you again, this time while you count backwards from 100 in threes (or if you hate numbers, while you say out loud as many different words as you can think of beginning with L).

Not so easy is it? You will find that at the very least you walked more slowly over the same distance. At worst you may have lost your balance – so take care with this exercise.

MOVING MORE
The three-week reset

The hardest part of any exercise, regardless of what type – walking, cycling, swimming, jogging, strength training or stretching – is always the same.

Starting.

Nothing is more difficult than making yourself begin. And that's where this three-week exercise plan comes in, providing you with detailed instructions on what to do each day, in collaboration with two of Britain's most inspiring and knowledgeable exercise experts: Dr Flaminia Ronca, associate professor of exercise neuroscience and programme director of Sport and Exercise Medical Sciences at UCL, and Dr Anne Elliott, senior lecturer in sports science at Middlesex University and a specialist in exercise for the middle-aged.

You're going to be doing just 15 minutes' exercise a day, plus a five-minute warm up. And not even every day – there are two rest days to give your body a chance to recover and assimilate the changes. (In the weekly programme we've devised, you'll see the rest days fall on Tuesday and Saturday, but as long as they are evenly spaced out, you can change the days to whichever suit you best).

As well as one strength or resistance exercise session each week, you'll be doing three cardio sessions: one at low intensity, one at medium intensity and one at high intensity. And each week there's a mobility/stretching session too, to keep both joints and muscles flexible. The sessions are the same every week, and in the following pages you will find detailed explanations of how to do each exercise.

As with the Fabulous Fibre food plan, this is a gentle, gradual introduction to improving your cardiovascular fitness, your power and strength, and how well your body functionally moves.

If you're consistent, you'll notice considerable changes both in your physical fitness and your general mood and wellbeing by the end of three weeks. At the end of the plan, you'll find Dr Ronca's mood questionnaire, which is an interesting and useful tool to help you find out which sort of exercise benefits your mood the most.

HOW FIT ARE YOU?

Before you start, it's important to gauge how fit you are now. Dr Elliott has compiled the following test. It's suitable for complete beginners, requires no equipment and takes only five minutes. Depending on how easy or difficult you find it, you can either begin the three-week plan straight away, or as an interim measure do Dr Elliott's exercise programme for beginners (see Appendix) before moving on to the three-week plan when you are ready.

Note: check with your doctor first if you have any concerns about starting any exercise programme.

A few safety points:
• Always do exercises in a space cleared of any obstacles.
• Always wear clothes that allow you to move freely in
  any direction.

- Always read the instructions carefully before attempting any exercise.
- Never push yourself to the point of pain. 'Feeling the burn' is not helpful.
- In these before and after tests, you are looking at how much *you* have improved rather than if you match up to some standard of how you 'should' do. When you are fitter, you can compare yourself to national averages.
- Don't forget to write down your test results so you can compare them four weeks later.

❶ Sit to stand test

This measures how strong your 'motion' muscles are (gluteals, hamstrings and quadriceps).

a. Place a dining chair with no arms next to a wall.

b. Sit down with one foot slightly in front of the other to help stability.

c. Cross your arms in front at your chest.

d. Count how many times you can stand up and sit down again in 30 seconds.

e. If this is too hard with your arms crossed, hold them to the side of you. Try not to use them.

❷ Chair seat and reach

This measures lower-body flexibility.

a. Sit on a dining chair with one leg bent and the other straight out in front of you with the heel on the floor.

b. Reach down the straight leg to your foot and measure how far your fingers go.

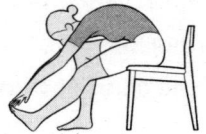

❸ Back scratch test

This measures upper-body flexibility.

a. Stand upright.

b. Stretch one hand back over your shoulder and down your back. With your other hand, reach round to the back from below. Can your hands meet? Check in a mirror how far apart they are.

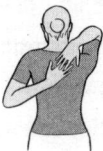

❹ Arm curl test

a. Sit in a dining chair and hold something such as a 500ml bottle of water in each hand or, if that is too heavy, a 400g tin of beans.

b. Keeping your back straight and against the chair, raise and lower the weights as many times as you can in 30 seconds. Move the arms from completely straight to as bent as your body allows.

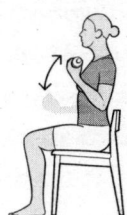

⑤ Walking upstairs

A functional movement that tests gait, lower-body strength, balance, core strength and muscle endurance. This is a subjective test.

• Walk up a flight of steps in your house, then turn and walk down again. Ask yourself these questions as you are doing it. Do not do anything that makes you feel unsafe.

• Am I standing upright as I walk up these stairs or am I bent forward? If so, by how much am I bent forward? (Demonstrates lower body strength.)

• Do I automatically hold the stair rail to help me? Am I using it to push against to help me up or do I use it for balance? (Demonstrates balance and strength.)

• How many steps can I do before I am breathing heavily? (Demonstrates cardiovascular strength)

• What am I doing to help myself get down the stairs safely? Do I twist towards the rail? (Demonstrates balance.)

• If I consciously try to walk up a few stairs upright without holding the rail, how many stairs can I do? (Demonstrates balance and core strength.)

Normal ranges:

Sit to stand test – 14–19 stand-up and sit-downs

Chair sit and reach – measurement between toes and fingertips **when foot is at 90 degrees** – 1–4in

Back scratch test – hands 2.5–10in apart

Arm curl test – 12–17 arm raises in 30 seconds.

If you found the exercises easy – great! You're ready to start the three-week plan. If you found them challenging, please don't worry. The important thing is that you've begun. Which means you've already started to get better. As mentioned above, you can do Dr Elliott's programme for beginners (see Appendix) first, if you prefer. It offers five simple exercises to do each day which take only 15 minutes. At the end of each week, take this test again. You'll be amazed, encouraged and motivated by how quickly your results change, and by how soon your mood and energy improve. Start the plan whenever you feel ready.

Note: both the three-week exercise plan and Dr Elliott's programme for beginners can be done at home and require no equipment other than a chair, a firm cushion or yoga block and two normal-sized cans of food or two small bottles of water (to be used as weights).

* * *

OK, time to get started. Here are explanations for how to do all the exercises. It's worth spending some time looking at them and trying them out, especially if you've never done them before, so that when you come to do the session, it really will take you only 15 minutes (plus the five-minute warm-up).

WARM-UP MOVES FOR STRENGTH EXERCISES

High knees

Inhale and bring your right knee as high up to your chest as possible. (If you want, put your left hand on a wall for balance and support.) Use your right arm to hug the knee closer as you begin to exhale, then keep exhaling as you lower the leg to the ground. Do this a few times, then do the same thing with your left leg (turning round if you want so that you can put your right hand on the wall).

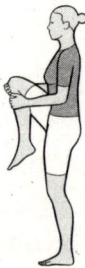

Jumping jacks

Stand with your feet slightly apart. Jump on the spot, swinging both arms above your head as you rise, and bringing them back down by your sides as you land.

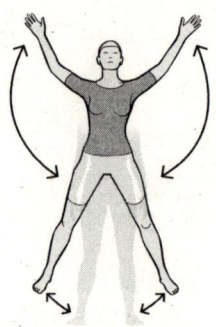

Hip rotations

With your left hand on the wall, lift and bend your right knee and point your toes. Move your knee slightly forward and then rotate it out to the right, down and back, activating your right hip as you form a small circle. Point your toes as you bring your foot down, and flex your foot as you bring it back up. Do this five times, then reverse the direction and do it five more times. Turn around and, with your right hand on the wall, go through the same movement with the left leg.

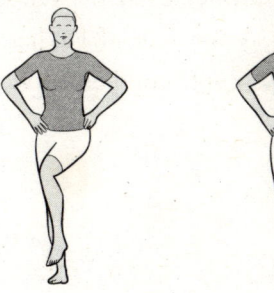

Leg swings

With your left hand on the wall, swing your right leg slowly forward and back eight times, keeping it straight. Then swing it out to the right eight times. Then with your right hand on the wall, do the same on the other side. Keep your hand on the wall for balance.

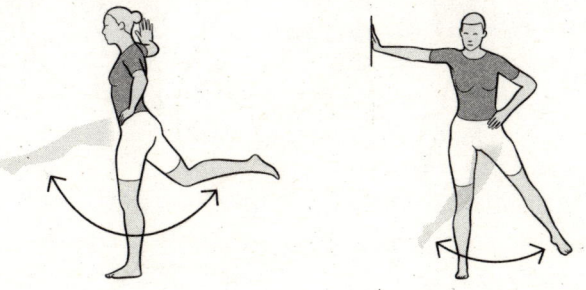

Plank

Lie flat on the floor on your stomach. Come up on to your elbows, with your forearms straight in front of you on the floor, palms down. Keep your legs straight and your feet flexed, so that your toes are touching the floor and the soles of your feet are facing straight out behind you. Engage your muscles – stomach, legs, glutes (buttocks) – and keep your back straight so that your bottom is tucked in rather than sticking up in the air. Remember to breathe!

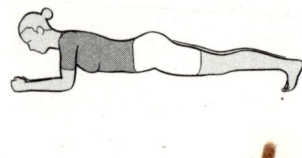

Arm windmills

Windmill your arms up in front of you, over your head, then out to the sides as you bring them back down eight times. Repeat in the opposite direction.

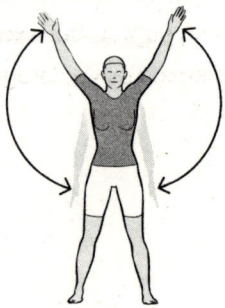 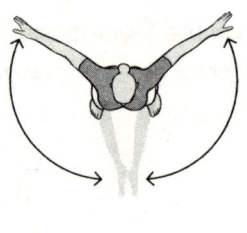

Arm swings

With your feet firmly planted on the ground and knees very slightly bent, keep your hips facing forward as you swing your arms up and to the left, so that your right arm comes across your chest. Do this eight times. Then switch direction. Don't go too fast or be too vigorous – this is quite a powerful exercise, especially if you do not have much upper-body mobility. Less is more at the beginning.

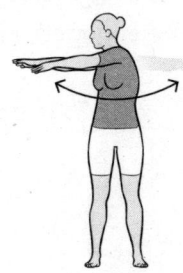

Jogging on the spot

This is just as it says on the tin: run on the spot. Again, don't go too quickly here if you are not used to this sort of exercise. And if you can't manage a whole minute, don't worry – do as much as you can, then stop. Keep a note of when you stop (for example, after 10 seconds). That way you can feel pleased as you progress to jogging for longer and longer each week.

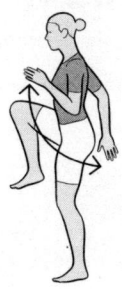

STRENGTH EXERCISES

Squat

Stand with your feet slightly wider than shoulder width apart, inhale, engage your core muscles and keep them engaged as you bend your knees and go down into a squat. Think about keeping as much weight as possible in your heels. When you've gone down as far as you can – imagine you are sitting on a chair – push down hard with your heels, keep your core engaged and slowly come back up, exhaling.

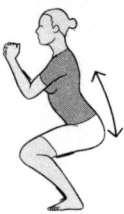

Kneeling press-up

Kneel on the floor and, keeping your feet flexed behind you, hinge forward to put your hands on the ground in front of you. Your arms should be straight, and your hands should be positioned directly beneath your shoulders. Lift your feet slightly and cross them at your ankles – you should now have only your knees and hands in contact with the floor. Keeping your spine long and without arching, look straight ahead and bend both your arms to lower your chest towards the floor. Then push back up to the starting position. If this is too much, do a wall press-up instead (see below).

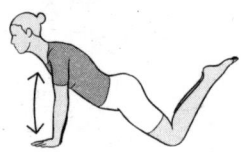

Wall press-up

Place your hands on the wall and move your feet back just far enough for your arms to be at parallel to the floor and shoulder height. Then bend at the elbows, looking straight ahead, keeping your spine long and without rounding your back, and bring your chest closer to the wall. Push back up into the starting position. The lower your hands and the further away your feet, the more difficult the exercise.

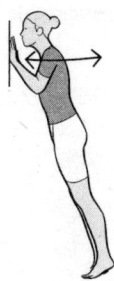

Plank with shoulder taps

Begin on your hands and knees with your elbows straight and hands on the floor shoulder width apart. Reach each foot back one at a time to form a 'plank'. You should have your core engaged and your back as straight as possible. Now lift your right hand off the floor and tap your left shoulder. Return your right hand to the floor and do the same with your left. Then repeat the tapping. If holding the plank is too much, stand up and, facing a wall, do the exercise in a wall press-up.

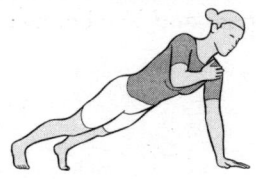

Lunge

If you are not used to doing lunges, start by doing them alongside a sofa so that you can put a hand down onto the sofa seat to help you balance. Stand with your feet a few inches apart. Engage your core muscles and pushing down firmly through your right heel, bend your right knee and slide your left leg behind you. Get down as low as you can, so that your left knee just kisses the floor – your core muscles should be engaged and your right knee positioned directly above your right ankle (i.e. at right angles to the floor). Pause for a moment, and then push down through your right heel to come back up, bringing your left foot back to its starting position. Repeat on the other side.

Side lunge

Stand with your feet slightly apart. Engage your core muscles. Keep your right foot where it is, and move your left leg out to the side as you bend your right knee. Pause. Keep your core muscles engaged. Then push down hard through your right heel as you slowly straighten your right leg and bring your left leg back to centre. *Don't go out too far with your leg* – if you're not used to this exercise, it's easy to strain your inner thighs, so take it gently. Repeat on the other side.

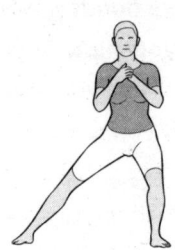

STRETCH AND MOBILITY EXERCISES

Warm-up stretch
Lie flat on your back, arms relaxed by your side. Put a hand on your stomach. Focus on expanding your abdomen as you inhale slowly, so that your hand moves slightly up. Then as you slowly exhale, feel your abdomen release and come back down. Take three calming breaths like this. Then inhale, sweep your arms overhead, tensing all your muscles, including those on your face, pointing your toes and stretching out your fingers. Exhale, and release.

Rocking
Lying on your back and engaging your core muscles, bend your knees, hug them in towards your chest and gently rock from side to side and then in small circles on your lower back and sacrum (the flat triangular bone at the base of your spine). Enjoy the movement, remembering to breathe, slowly.

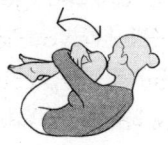

Cat cow
Come on to all fours, with your hands positioned beneath your shoulders and knees below your hips. As you inhale, let your stomach drop down and gently tilt your pelvis back as you curve your spine, vertebra by vertebra, from the base to the top, expanding your chest as you do so. Keep your neck long and relaxed. Then, as you exhale, drop your chin to your chest, pull

your stomach muscles in and arch your spine, vertebra by vertebra, in the opposite direction, upwards (like an angry cat).

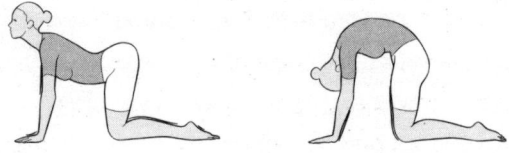

Neck rolls

Stand with your feet shoulder width apart. Drop your chin to your chest and roll your right ear slowly towards your right shoulder, then drop your head gently back and roll your left ear round towards your left shoulder, before rolling your chin back to the centre of your chest. Repeat twice then switch direction. You cannot go too slowly – the slower the better.

Now drop your right ear towards your right shoulder and rest your right hand gently on top of your head to increase the neck stretch. Don't push, just let the weight of your hand increase the pressure slightly. If you can, bend your left elbow and bring your left arm behind and between your shoulder blades with the palm facing out. Hold for five slow inhales and exhales. Repeat on the other side.

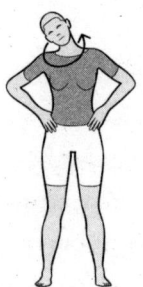 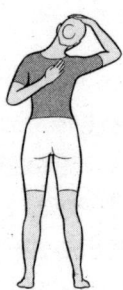

Cross-legged sitting with crossed arms

Come into a cross-legged position with your right leg in front of your left. If it's uncomfortable, sit on cushions or a yoga block. Hold your arms out in front of you, then cross them over to give yourself a hug, with your left arm on top. If you find this too difficult, rest each hand on the opposite shoulder. Feel the stretch across the tops of your shoulders and upper back. Hold for five slow inhales and exhales. Still sitting cross-legged, and keeping your arms as they are, fold forward and hold for five more slow inhales and exhales. Staying forward, release your arms and bring them to the floor in front of you, or as close to the floor as possible. If they don't reach the floor, you can rest them on cushions. Hold for five more slow breaths.

Slowly come back up. Switch legs so that now you are cross-legged with your left leg in front, then cross the right arm on top of the left. Repeat. Lastly, uncross your legs, bend them at the knee and then, with your hands on the floor just behind you, and both feet on the ground, slowly bring both legs across to the right and then to the left in a windshield wiper motion. Do this several times to release your hips.

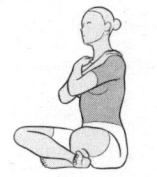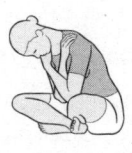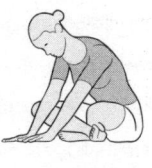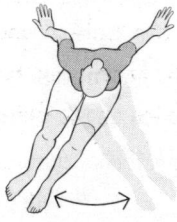

Supported squat

You will need to hold onto something solid for this exercise, such as the edge of a sink. With your feet flat on the floor and together, hold onto the edge of the sink with both hands and slowly bend your knees to come down towards the floor. Keep your knees as far apart as possible and drop your chin to your chest. Aim to round your spine as much as possible and to come down as low as possible. Then hold for five slow inhales and exhales, bouncing very gently. Push down hard through your heels and engage your core as you slowly come back up. Take two slow inhales and exhales.

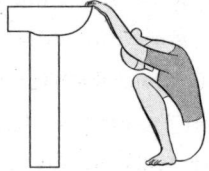

Supported bridge

You will need a couple of firm cushions or a yoga block. Lie on your back, bend your knees and walk your feet in towards your glutes. Push down hard through your heels to lift your bottom and place the yoga block or equivalent under your sacrum. It is important that the block goes here and not under your lumbar region or lower back. Have the block horizontal, with its largest, widest side flat on the floor. You can keep your knees bent and only when and if that feels comfortable should you try gently straightening your legs. Keep your arms out to the sides to start with and then try bringing them overhead, but only if that feels comfortable. You should feel a mild compression in the spine, and a pleasurable stretch along the entire front of the body. If it's painful, go back to knees bent. Relax as much as you can – it is easy to tense up here, and not at all necessary, as your body is fully supported by the floor and the block. Breathe slowly and comfortably. Then bend your knees and walk your feet back in, remove the block and slowly come down vertebra by vertebra.

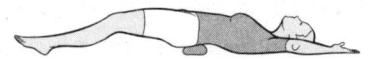

Supine spinal twist

Lying on your back, spread your arms out to either side and let your knees fall gently over to the left. Try to keep both shoulders on the floor. If your right shoulder is far off the ground, you can put a pillow or cushion underneath for support. If your knees don't reach the ground or if there is a gap between them, again, use a block or cushion. You should feel a stretch along the right-hand side of your body from your toes to your arms. The higher you bring your right arm (keeping it on the floor), the more stretch you'll feel. Go slowly and don't push it. Your body will open up slowly over time. Breathe slowly and comfortably for 10 breaths.

Slowly come back to centre, rock gently, then bring your arms out to the sides again and let your knees fall gently to the right. Hold for 10 breaths. Come back to centre, hug your knees, rock gently and then rest on the mat in whatever position feels comfortable for a minute or two.

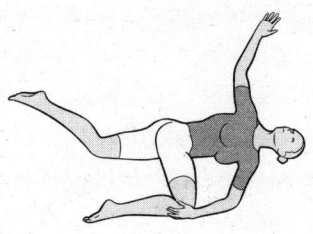

* * *

Now you know how to do the exercises, let's begin! Remember that you're going to be doing just 15 minutes' exercise a day, plus a five-minute warm up. The sessions are the same every week and include two rest days to give your body a chance to recover.

YOUR WEEK AT A GLANCE

SUNDAY
Medium intensity – 20 mins

MONDAY
Strength session – 20 mins

TUESDAY
Rest day

WEDNESDAY
High intensity – 3 × 1 min sets

THURSDAY
Stretching and mobility – 20 mins

FRIDAY
Low intensity / recovery session – 20 mins

SATURDAY
Rest day

SUNDAY
Medium intensity – 20 minutes
This session is designed in collaboration with Dr Ronca and Dr Tom Gurney, lecturer in exercise physiology at UCL, to work around the lactate threshold, also known as the anaerobic threshold (the point at which the body switches from aerobic to anaerobic metabolism and begins to burn stored sugars for energy). It helps improve our ability to sustain vigorous intensities for prolonged periods.

Warm-up – 5 minutes
High knees × 10
Jumping jacks × 10
Hip rotations × 10 each side
Leg swings × 8 each side
Plank: hold for 20 seconds – and remember to breathe!
    Rest 20 seconds, then repeat
Arm windmills × 8 each side
Arm swings × 8 each side. Remember to go slowly
Jogging on the spot (1 minute – or for as long as you can)

Choose one of the following:
5 minutes' speed walking, going into a 10-minute jog
5 minutes' cycling, going into 10 minutes' fast cycling
5 minutes' speed walking on the flat, going into 10 minutes' speed walking up hill.

The aim here is to get your heart rate up first, to the point where you can hold a conversation, even though you feel a bit breathless while doing so – on a scale from 1 to 10, where 1 is super easy and 10 is all-out, your perceived effort should be around 5 or 6. Then, after 5 minutes, the idea is to increase the intensity so that you can't speak more than a few words and your effort is 7 or 8. It should feel uncomfortable but just about manageable.

If you can't manage the entire 10 minutes at the more intense level, don't worry. Do as much as you can, then go back to speed walking or slower cycling. Pick up the pace again when you feel able. As the weeks go by, you will find it gets easier.

MONDAY
Strength session – 20 minutes

Warm-up as before (5 minutes)
Do three sets of the following, resting for 1 minute between each set and for 20 seconds between each exercise:
Plank with shoulder taps (30 seconds)
Kneeling press-up: (30 seconds)
Squats (30 seconds)
Lunges (30 seconds)
Side lunges (30 seconds)

On the lunges, keep your core engaged throughout and don't forget to breathe! Remember: if you are not used to doing lunges, start by doing them alongside a seat to help you balance. On the side lunges, don't go out too far with your leg on either side, as you can easily strain your inner thigh muscles. Slower, and less, is better as you gradually build strength, mobility and flexibility.

TUESDAY: rest day

WEDNESDAY
High intensity – 3 × 1 minute sets

Warm-up as before (5 minutes)
Choose one of the following:
Rope skipping, fast running, all-out cycling or fast high knees
    for 1 minute
Rest 3 minutes
Repeat the exercise for 1 minute
Rest 3 minutes
Repeat for 1 more minute
Rest

THURSDAY
Mobility/stretching – 20 minutes

Warm-up stretch (× 3)
Rocking × 5 in each direction
Cat cow × 5
Neck rolls × 3 in each direction; right ear to right shoulder,
    5 × slow breaths; left ear to left shoulder, 5 × slow breaths;
    fold forward chin to chest, × 5 slow breaths
Cross-legged sitting with crossed arms, 5 × slow breaths upright,
    5 × slow breaths leaning forward, × 5 slow breaths arms out
    in front, each side
Supported squats × 3.
Supported bridge 10 × slow breaths
Rocking 3 × slow breaths
Supine spinal twist 10 × breaths each side

FRIDAY
Low-intensity recovery session – 15 minutes
This is a recovery session, which builds endurance while also helping you recover.

Warm-up as before (5 minutes)
Choose from:
Brisk walking, jogging or cycling and keep to a fairly easy pace. It shouldn't be a stroll but it shouldn't be uncomfortable – your effort should be around 4. It should be possible for you to hold a conversation for the entire 15 minutes, even though you might prefer not to.

SATURDAY: rest day

* * *

Keep a note of how you feel at the end of each week, and how you found each day's exercise. Mark any that you found difficult, so that by the end of the three weeks you can see how much you've progressed.

Of course, you can continue this plan after the three weeks is up. I very much hope you will! And remember that once an exercise starts to feel easy, you can take it up a level, either by adding weight, using dumbbells – start light (2kg in each hand) and work your way up – or by increasing the repetitions, or both.

HOW TO LEARN TO LOVE EXERCISE

If you're a reluctant exerciser, I sympathise. I was once one too. And if someone had told me I had to start going to a gym several times a week, I would have run a mile (well, I wouldn't have been able to run even a quarter of a mile back then – but you know what I mean!). In the end, I found my way into exercise gradually, doing little bits here and there as a way to strengthen my ailing back and rid myself of pain. And here's the thing: little bits here and there are the building blocks of a little bit more here and there. It makes you feel good. And before you know it, you are consciously building movement into your everyday life which helps you become fitter and more mobile almost effortlessly. Small decisions add up, over time, to big change.

So: if you don't live somewhere really remote and don't have very small children, walk to the shops or take public transport instead of driving (unless you're doing a big supermarket shop, of course). Buy a rucksack if you don't already have one, and put smaller bits and pieces of shopping into that.

Think about getting off the bus or train one stop earlier in the evening, and walk one stop further in the morning. It's a lovely way to start and end your commute. At lunchtime, get outside and walk, even if it's just for 10 minutes (do it after you've eaten if possible – it's one of the best ways to lower your blood sugar. The same applies after your evening meal). If you're working from home and therefore don't have to commute, get out for a walk in the morning and evening anyway.

In public buildings, always take the stairs rather than the lift (unless it's a skyscraper). Walk up escalators rather than just standing there. When making or receiving phone calls, walk around (better still, go outside to do so). Walking whenever you can will soon become a habit, one which benefits both your body and your mind.

I mentioned earlier that exercise releases dopamine, the same pleasurable feeling that people get from certain narcotics. And just as addicts crave their next hit, the same will happen to you with exercise. All you have to do is find the thing you most enjoy doing. Because if you find it fun you'll be more likely to do the hardest part – start. It really doesn't matter what it is – dancing, pickleball, climbing, swimming, roller blading, hiking, running, tennis... There are so many forms of exercise and ALL of them will improve your mood, your fitness, your health and, if you do them enough, ultimately your longevity. What's not to love about that?

GOOD BALANCE

Good balance is important at any age, but as you get older it becomes crucial. According to statistics from the Institute of Public Care at Oxford Brookes university, one in three people over the age of 65 will have a fall.

Yoga and Pilates classes are terrific for improving balance, as they both involve balancing postures, such as tree or warrior 3 in yoga or the various types of lunges in Pilates.

But you can also improve your balance every day at home. Try balancing on one foot for one minute while you brush your teeth, switching to the other foot halfway through. Start with one hand on the sink for support and gradually lift it for longer and longer periods until you can balance for an entire minute on each leg. (And when you've cracked that, try it with your eyes closed!).

Once you feel you have good balance, you can also try doing one-legged squats while brushing your teeth: with your right foot pressing firmly into the floor, bend the knee and lift your left leg behind you. Then repeat on the other side.

HOW TO IMPROVE FUNCTIONAL MOVEMENT OF LEGS, SPINE AND HIPS

If you ask a five-year-old to get up from a cross-legged position on the floor without using their hands they will do so effortlessly, without even thinking. But if you try it yourself you may find it rather more difficult, maybe even impossible.

However, the ability to do so is a key indicator of longevity and general fitness. It requires both strength and mobility in your legs, back and hips. I was shocked, when I tried it myself a couple of years ago, to find that I couldn't do it without using my hands – even after years of running, yoga and pilates. My old injury meant that despite all that, my lower back was still weak, and as for my hips – they had barely any functional mobility at all.

So I began doing the following exercises every morning, thanks to Juliet and Kelly Starrett's excellent book, *Built To Move*. After a few months, I found I could finally get up from the floor without using my hands – not effortlessly, but I could do it. I still do the exercises first thing every morning, and have come to really enjoy them.

- Sit cross-legged, right leg in front, spine straight (2 minutes).
- Now sit with your left leg in front (2 minutes).
- Bring both legs straight out in front of you (2 minutes).

- Hug your right knee in and hold it as close as you can to your chest, keeping your left leg and your spine straight (2 minutes).
- Hug your left knee in as close to your chest as possible, with your right leg straight (2 minutes).
- Bend your right knee at 90 degrees flat on the floor, so your right foot is in line with your left hip, then bend your left knee and bring it behind you (2 minutes); repeat on the other side.
- Now go back to sitting cross-legged and stand up. Repeat three more times.

LIFELINE: HOW TO USE AN OLD BROOM HANDLE TO OPEN YOUR SHOULDERS AND CHEST AND RELEASE TENSION

This is one of the best exercises there is to release tension in your chest and shoulders from sitting. I do it every day.

Stand with your feet hip width apart and keep a microbend in your knees. Hold the broom handle horizontally in front of you, hands a few inches wider than hip width apart. Inhale and with straight arms lift the handle up above your head. As you exhale, start to bring it behind your head until you reach a point of resistance (which may not be very far at all). You will start to feel a deep stretch across your upper chest and the backs of your shoulders. Then inhale to bring the handle back over your head to the starting point. Go slowly and don't force it – many of us are extremely tight in these areas. As your shoulders become more flexible, you will be able to bring the handle further behind your head.

Now take it a step further, if you can. Bring the broom handle above your head, then inhale and, keeping your hips and head facing forwards, twist from the waist slowly to the right, bringing the left end of the broom slowly down and diagonally towards your right hip and keeping your right arm up. From there begin to twist slowly back to centre, bringing your left arm down in front of your left hip, then your right arm down in front of your right hip, so that now the broom handle is horizontal in front of you at hip level. Now twist to the left, bringing first your left arm up, then your right, so that now you are twisted left from your thoracic spine, with your hips facing forward, and the broom handle held above your head to the left. Keeping the broom handle above your head, come back slowly to centre. Repeat the process in the opposite direction. Repeat five times on each side.

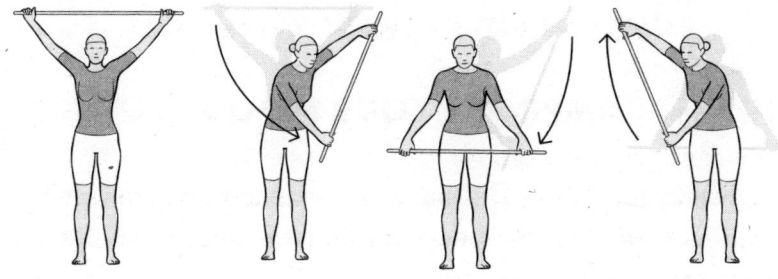

CHANGE THE WAY YOU SIT

If you spend most of your day sitting at a desk – as I have done for more than 30 years – it's time to take action. Because unless you have a posture that wouldn't be out of place in an episode of *Bridgerton*, it's likely you spend much of your time with rounded, hunched shoulders and your pelvis pushed back. Sitting like this for hours is ruining our lower backs, shoulders, necks and hips and is one of the main reasons we are in such pain as we age.

There are various strategies that will help. Set an alarm on your phone and get up to walk around for a few minutes every hour. Do supported squats (see mobility exercises in the exercise plan) as often as you can throughout the day. Invest in a lumbar support to tie around the back of your chair – it will support your lower back and help correct the position of your pelvis and spine. Also aim to do shoulder shrugs with shoulder rotations or the broom handle exercise as often as you can, perhaps in one of your mini breaks each hour. The key is to do these small things every day, frequently. It only takes a few minutes, which you can easily build into your day's work, and you will be amazed at the difference it makes.

IMPROVE YOUR MOOD

Fascinating research by Dr Ronca[12] shows that the type of exercise that lifts your mood best depends on what sort of personality you have.

———

12 Her study (Body fat predictive of acute effects of exercise on prefrontal hemodynamics and speed. *Neuropsychologia*, 2024 – https://pubmed.ncbi.nlm.nih. gov/38340963/) involved 132 people. Each was given an online questionnaire to rate their stress levels, and also a psychometric test to determine which of the Big Five personality traits they showed (extraversion, conscientiousness, agreeableness, neuroticism and openness). The volunteers were then divided into groups – a control group, which just maintained their normal lifestyle, and an intervention group, which followed an 8-week cycling and strength training plan programme.

In week 1 the intervention group were asked to rate their enjoyment of each training session from 1–7. After 8 weeks, all the participants, from both groups, completed the online stress questionnaire again.

'Personality, birth sex and fitness level all influence which forms of activity we enjoy the most, and which ones boost our mood the most,' she says. 'For example, we've seen that while most people's mood improves after either strength training or running, men's mood typically improves more than women's mood after a strength session [surprised?], but women's mood improves more than men's mood after running. In another example, extraversion predicts greater enjoyment of high-intensity sessions.'

It's a really good idea to get a notebook and jot down each day how you feel before and after each session, which exercises you enjoyed and which you didn't, and to try to give an overall mood/ stress score for each session. Score yourself from 1–7, where 1 is not at all, 4 is neutral and 7 is very much, in answer to these four questions: how sleepy do you feel right now? How energised do you feel? How happy do you feel? How sad do you feel?

At the end of three weeks you will have a useful record – not only of how you've progressed physically but in terms of your mood and stress too. Remember that not all days are the same. Some days a particular session might benefit you more than others, and that's perfectly normal. Keep tracking consistently throughout the three weeks so you can get a more comprehensive picture of how your mood responds to the various sessions.

Dr Ronca's study found that just 15 minutes of yoga are enough to improve our mood. But what improves mood most is 30 minutes of moderate to vigorous aerobic exercise, for example, running or cycling, compared to stretching, yoga, strength training and either light cycling or HIIT (high-intensity interval training). They also found that people's fitness level (or lack of fitness) did not affect their mood – the change in mood came from doing the activity itself, regardless of how fit or not they were.

Why I think the best forms of yoga are Bikram and yin

Yoga has wonderful benefits if taught correctly in a class which is suitable for your level, rather than in a class where you could injure yourself either because the pace is too fast for you and/or where the teacher isn't checking to see that you're doing the postures correctly.

It can be extremely grounding and mentally calming and it will certainly improve your co-ordination, balance, suppleness and mobility.

But, if you are middle-aged, unused to exercise and with limited or weak upper and lower body strength, my advice is to supplement it with weight training and cardio exercise. Also, beware the cult of 'Insta yoga'. The real purpose of yoga is breath control and finding your inner calm. It should never be about showing off.

My yoga preferences are Bikram and yin. For those who don't know, Bikram involves a set sequence of 26 postures over 90 minutes, done in a studio heated to 40 degrees C. It works your heart and also your mental resilience, as half the battle for a beginner is resisting the urge to leave the room because of the heat.

Yin is slower-paced and more meditative, and involves holding passive poses, sometimes for several minutes. It is taught in many yoga studios and also online.

I've been doing both for years, and have found that they are the forms in which you are least likely to injure yourself. They are both suitable for any level, and have considerable benefits, not least in relieving depression and anxiety.

A 2023 clinical trial led by Massachussetts General Hospital randomly divided depressed adults into two groups, one assigned two 90-minute sessions of Bikram hot yoga a week, and one told that they were on a waiting list so did not receive any treatment.

After just eight weeks, nearly half of the adults recruited to do two 90-minute Bikram sessions a week had seen such a dramatic improvement in their symptoms that they were no longer classed as depressed. And most of those taking part in the hot yoga said the severity of their symptoms had eased by at least 50 per cent, compared with just 6 per cent of the control group.

But you don't have to be depressed to enjoy Bikram. It is fabulous for all aspects of health, involving cardio, balance, stretching and the ability to control your breath and with it your mind. After a while you come to love the sweat and the 40 degree heat... truly!

As for yin yoga (full disclosure: I teach yin myself), various studies show that it reduces anxiety and stress[1] in such a way as to be beneficial against heart disease. It is slow, involving long-held postures, almost all while sitting or lying down, and is quite transformative for both body and mind.

---

1 The effect of yin yoga intervention on state and trait anxiety during the COVID-19 pandemic. *Front. Psych.*, 2024 – www.ncbi.nlm.nih.gov/pmc/articles/PMC10973109/

Impact of a Yin Yoga and meditation intervention on pharmacy faculty and student well-being. *J. Amer. Pharm. Assoc.*, 2021 – www.sciencedirect.com/science/article/abs/pii/S1544319121001904

Five-week yin yoga-based interventions decreased plasma adrenomedullin and increased psychological health in stressed adults. *PLOS One*, 2018 – www.researchgate.net/publication/326485473_

4
RESTING MORE DEEPLY

How well do you sleep?

❶ Do you often have difficulty falling asleep when you get into bed? If yes, go to question 2. If no, go to question 3.

❷ How long does it usually take you to fall asleep?
   a. 10–20 minutes;
   b. 30–45 minutes
   c. About an hour
   d. Well over an hour, sometimes 2 or 3

❸ Do you often wake up in the middle of the night and have difficulty going back to sleep?
   If yes, go to question 4. If no, go to question 5.

❹ How long does it take you on average to go back to sleep when you wake in the night?
   a. More than an hour
   b. Between 30 minutes and an hour
   c. 20–30 minutes
   d. 10 minutes or less

5 **What do you do to go back to sleep when you wake in the night?**

a. Nothing, I just relax and wait to fall asleep again

b. I go to the loo or have some water

c. I look at my phone to see the time and then start worrying that if I don't get back to sleep soon I'll be really tired in the morning

d. If I can't get back to sleep I get up and listen to a podcast or read a book in another room

6 **Do you snore?**

7 **What time do you have your last coffee of the day?**

a. Around 3–4pm

b. After my evening meal

c. 12–1pm

d. 11am or before

8 **How much light is there in your bedroom when the curtains or blinds are drawn?**

a. A little

b. None – it's very dark

c. Quite a bit, especially as it gets light towards morning

d. Lots

9 **How do you usually feel when you wake up?**

a. A bit tired but OK

b. Thirsty and/or with a headache

c. Very tired and wishing I could sleep longer

d. Refreshed and ready to go

10 **How many hours' sleep do you usually get a night?**
   a. 8–9
   b. 6–8
   c. More than 9
   d. Less than 6

Answers
1 Score 1 for yes / 3 for no
2 a.1   **b.**2   **c.**3   **d.**4
3 Score 2 for **yes** / 1 for **no**
4 a.4   **b.**3   **c.**2   **d.**1
5 a.1   **b.**3   **c.**4   **d.**2
6 Score 2 for **yes** / 1 for **no**
7 a.3   **b.**4   **c.**2   **d.**1
8 a.2   **b.**1   **c.**3   **d.**4
9 a.2   **b.**3   **c.**4   **d.**1
10 a.1   **b.**2   **c.**3   **d.**4

Scores
14 or less: Congratulations – you sleep very well
14–22: Your sleep isn't perfect but is more or less OK
23–30: You don't sleep very well at all
31–40: You sleep very poorly – and must be shattered!

* * *

You probably don't need me to tell you how important sleep is. Barely a week goes by without a new study telling us how much of it we need, and there is a huge and profitable industry devoted to selling us products to help us, from beds and bedding to gadgets that measure everything from the actual time spent in the various phases of sleep to whether we snore and how we regulate our body temperature.

And all, generally, for good reason. No matter how well we eat or how long we run or how many weights we lift at the gym, without sleep, our bodies can't process that good work effectively. Sleep allows the body and brain to recover and is absolutely key to slowing down the ageing process.

For huge numbers of us, however, getting enough quality sleep at night is a struggle. The latest data shows that around one in three people in the West have problems with sleep at least one or two nights a week. And one in 10 say it's a routine problem for them that happens more often than not.

So before we go any further, let me give you two pieces of good news.

The first is that it is entirely possible to get your sleep back on track, using no medication whatsoever. The methods I am going to show you in the three-week reset plan work even for people who have had trouble sleeping for years. They are simple, scientifically proven, and used by some of the world's top sleep clinics.

The second is that there is a back-up mode of sleep, called yoga nidra (yogic sleep), or deep rest – by which I mean being able to switch off and put yourself into a state of deep, meditative rest at any point during the day when you are stressed or tired, or just not feeling your best. This will leave you feeling refreshed and restored even if you slept badly the night before. Indeed, in terms of the benefits to your body, it is said by many who do it regularly to be equivalent to a few hours' actual sleep. Imagine that…

Although there are no studies to prove this (yet – research is limited but scientific interest in this area is growing rapidly), a clinical trial in 2022[1] that measured some of the electrophysiological channels that characterise sleep found that after two weeks, participants who were new to yoga nidra demonstrated delta wave changes, similar to those found in sleep, even though they were awake. And a review[2] in 2021 of 50 studies shows there are remarkable benefits to be gained from regularly practising deep rest, among them reduced blood pressure, improved heart rate variability (see box on p189), improved regulation of hormones and blood glucose and a 65 per cent increase in dopamine.

A session of deep rest takes just 20–30 minutes to do (although you can do it for longer) and is foolproof. And I suggest that if you are someone who finds it difficult to get a good night's sleep, you skip the next section and go straight to page 170 which explains how to do it. One session is all it takes to feel re-energised and the more you do it, the better it gets. After a few sessions, you will feel less panicky about sleep and more confident of being able to get at least some restorative rest every day in 30 minutes or less. And you will then be able to embark on the three-week sleep reset in a calmer and more hopeful frame of mind.

SLEEP ANXIETY

Perhaps the worst effect of not getting enough sleep – aside from feeling exhausted – is the anxiety it induces. There was a time when it was clever to boast about how little sleep you needed. The

---

1 Electrophysiological evidence of local sleep during yoga nidra practice. *Front Neurol.* 2022 – pmc.ncbi.nlm.nih.gov/articles/PMC9315270/
2 The Origin and Clinical Relevance of Yoga Nidra. *Sleep Vigil.*, 2022 – pubmed. ncbi.nlm.nih.gov/35496325/

world admired Margaret Thatcher for getting by on just four hours a night and many of the world's most successful politicians and business leaders followed her example. In the 80s, 90s and early 2000s, the message was clear: sleep was for wimps. The way to get ahead was to spend as many hours as possible working.

Now we know better. Mrs T was one of the most influential figures of her age, with a brilliant mind. She also died with Alzheimer's. And we now know that *chronic, consistent* lack of sleep increases your chances of most of the major diseases, from dementia – the biggest killer in the UK in 2023 – to heart disease, stroke, diabetes and cancer. Oh, and it will probably also make you fat, by altering your appetite-regulating hormones, causing you to feel hungrier and be more likely to reach for sugary, fatty food.

However, don't panic! The clue is in those two words: chronic and consistent. Because as Dr Michael Grandner, one of the world's top sleep clinicians, points out, if we were that sensitive to lack of sleep, the human race would have died out long ago.

It's not that the risks of insufficient sleep aren't real; it's that they need to be taken in context.

A good analogy he likes to use to reassure people is eating pizza. Sleep is related to heart disease, diabetes and Alzheimer's, just like pizza is.

'But if you eat a pizza today, you're not going to get diabetes tomorrow,' he says. 'It's not about one pizza. It's not about a week's worth of pizza or even a month's worth of pizza. It's about the pattern. If sleep weren't flexible, we wouldn't have made it this far. So with sleep, it's not about tonight. It's not about a week, it's not even about one year. It's about a whole lifestyle pattern. One spate of bad sleep is not going to give you dementia.'

Nevertheless, even with Dr Grandner's reassurance firmly in mind, the facts about sleep are sobering.

As Matthew Walker, professor of neuroscience at Berkeley and an expert in sleep science, says, being deprived of just one night's good sleep causes much more physical and mental damage than the equivalent loss of exercise or good diet.

We live in a society that is constantly 'on', where being busy is seen as a symbol of success. We have forgotten how to do nothing, so much so that most people find it incredibly difficult even to relax, let alone have a good night's sleep.

Professor Walker says that a third of us – one in three people in the UK – don't get the recommended 7–9 hours' sleep a night. The average night's sleep in the UK is six hours 49 minutes; in the US, six hours 43 minutes. The consequences of regularly getting less than seven hours' sleep are enough to give anyone nightmares. Professor Walker points out that there have been more than 20 large-scale studies, tracking millions of people over many years, which all report the same thing: the shorter someone sleeps, the shorter their life.

In three large cohort studies, for example, ranging from 83,000 to 1.1 million people, sleeping 5 hours or less increased mortality risk, from all causes, by roughly 15 per cent.[3]

Another[4] showed that if you are 45 or older, sleeping less than six hours a night means you are at three times the risk of having a heart attack or stroke in your lifetime, while one night of modest sleep reduction – even just one or two hours less – can increase blood pressure significantly.

Furthermore, regularly sleeping less than six hours a night means you are three times more likely to have calcification of the arteries.

---

3 Sleep disorders and sleep deprivation: an unmet public health problem. *Nat. Acad. Press*, 2006 – www.ncbi.nlm.nih.gov/books/NBK19961/
4 Short sleep duration and incident coronary artery calcification. *JAMA*, 2008 – https://pubmed.ncbi.nlm.nih.gov/19109114/

You are more prone to Alzheimer's and dementia,[5] and also to eating more,[6] as your appetite hormones – leptin, for satiety, and ghrelin, for hunger – are no longer properly regulated. Leptin decreases and ghrelin increases, meaning you feel hungrier.

In one trial,[7] sleep-deprived participants ate 300 more calories during the next day than the well-slept control group.

Contrast all that with the benefits of a good night's sleep:

- Our brain is enriched, meaning we learn better, memorise better and make logical decisions.
- It optimises our memory storage facility. In a fascinating study using MRI scans, Professor Walker and his team were able to observe which part of the brain participants were retrieving their memories from, both before and after sleep. Before sleep, the memories were stored in what Professor Walker calls the 'short-term storage site' in the hippocampus. But the next morning, after a full night's sleep, the memories had moved and were now being retrieved from the neocortex, a long-term storage site for fact-based memories. This cycle repeats every night, meaning each day's memories are safely stowed away overnight, freeing short-term storage capacity for new learning the next day.
- Our emotional brain circuits recalibrate while we dream, so that we can face whatever the day throws at us more calmly. During the rapid eye movement (REM) phase when we dream, which comes in the second half of our sleep, painful memories are soothed. Research shows that the more we

---

5 www.alzheimersresearchuk.org/news/dreaming-of-a-world-without-dementia
6 Metabolic consequences of sleep and sleep loss. *Sleep Med.*, 2015 – pmc.ncbi. nlm.nih.gov/articles/PMC4444051
7 news.uchicago.edu/story/sleep-loss-boosts-hunger-and-high-calorie-food-choices

dream about a trauma we've experienced, such as a painful divorce, the faster we recover emotionally – the dream allows the brain to process it. But not only that: dreaming also allows our brains to combine past and present knowledge, helping us be creative and come up with solutions to difficult problems.

- Our immune system is rebalanced, together with our blood sugar and insulin levels.
- It helps to maintain the microbiome in our gut – the bacteria which not only improve our digestion but also our brain function – and regulates our cardiovascular system.

Given all that, who wouldn't want to get the best sleep possible, every night? As Bryan Johnson, the billionaire who is spending millions optimising his longevity and is fanatical about sleep, points out: 'Sleep deprivation makes hard things feel impossible. High-quality sleep makes seemingly impossible things doable.'

Although perhaps most of us are not prepared to go to quite the same extremes as Bryan in our quest for a good night's sleep. His X post in July 2023 still makes me laugh:

'What I share on first dates:
11am dinner
8.30pm bed'

He then lists another 10 or so requirements, from 'u sleep alone' to 'scheduled sex' and 'no pillow talk' before his pay off: 'Unsure why I'm single'.

But for him it works. He sleeps eight and a half hours a night and says he has never felt better. However, you don't have to be in bed by 8.30pm every night to achieve a great night's sleep. By that I mean a solid 7.5–8.5 hours every night, from which you wake up feeling refreshed and ready to go. If you are one of these fortunate people, I suggest you skip the next few pages. Anyone else, from intermittently poor sleepers to full-on insomniacs, read on!

IS IT ACTUALLY INSOMNIA?

The broad definition of insomnia is difficulty sleeping. But for insomnia to be clinically relevant, it has to meet the criteria known by sleep scientists as $3 \times 30 \times 3$: it has to happen three nights a week or more; last for 30 minutes or more; and have been a problem for three months or more. It also has to be causing you difficulties during the day, for example, with work because of difficulty staying awake or concentrating, or relationship issues because you are moody or bad-tempered.

Insomnia can happen at any time of night. It could be that you have trouble falling asleep, or that you fall asleep easily but wake in the middle of the night and then can't get back to sleep; or that you sleep quite well until quite far through the night but then wake up an hour or more before you need to and can't get back to sleep.

Incidentally, if you suffer from a lack of sleep, rather than have difficulty sleeping, then it is not insomnia; it is sleep deprivation (although a person can have both). A shift worker who struggles to fall asleep in the middle of the day after their night shift ends does not have an insomnia problem but a circadian rhythm issue (see p168). A coffee drinker who likes to have a cup not long before bed and then can't sleep doesn't have insomnia: their lack of sleep is due to a chemical. Someone who binged on a box set until 2am despite having to get up for work at 7am also does not have insomnia, and nor does the new parent whose baby is keeping them awake most of the night. They are all suffering from sleep deprivation.

That said, all these examples, if repeated often enough, may well *lead* to insomnia, as I explain below…

WHAT'S HAPPENING IN YOUR BRAIN WHEN YOU CAN'T SLEEP

As Dr Michael Grandner, who runs the Sleep Clinic at the University of Arizona puts it, after a while it doesn't matter what originally caused your lack of sleep. It could have started because you had a young baby who woke frequently in the night, or because you used always to have a coffee not long before bed, or because you had a period when you were worried about money or a future event like exams or a wedding.

The point is that, whatever the cause, if the insomnia continues, eventually the lack of sleep itself becomes a habit, with a momentum all of its own.

Dr Grandner (whose clinic has a 90 per cent success rate treating patients with sleep problems) is a strong advocate for CBT-I (cognitive behavioural therapy for insomnia) for sleep problems, and has two techniques which he says are 'shockingly successful – even if you've had insomnia for decades'. These are stimulus control and time restricted sleeping, and they are useful for anyone who has trouble falling asleep, even if their sleep problem doesn't actually qualify as chronic insomnia.

Dr Grandner explains it to patients like this: 'CBT-I is based on the principle that whatever caused your insomnia initially is largely irrelevant. Think of a ball rolling down a hill. Something pushed the ball to make it roll down the hill. The push was the problem.

But once the ball is rolling, the push becomes irrelevant. The real problem at this point is gravity, because the ball doesn't require more pushing to keep rolling.

'That's what happens with insomnia. And in fact, it starts even before the push. It starts with the actual hill itself. We all have a hill. Yours may be steep, mine may be shallow, everyone's is a little bit different. For some people it requires a lot to get that ball rolling. For others, the ball starts rolling with barely a push at all. Some people are more reactive than others. Some people are more sensitive to noise or whatever. The hill is what we call your *predisposition* – which, though important, is not really changeable.

'The push comes next. It's what we call the *precipitating* factor – the thing that gets the ball rolling, or which starts keeping you awake instead of asleep. This factor may or may not be preventable, but it is usually what people focus on. It's anything that increases activation in your mind or your body, which could theoretically lead you to be awake when you want to be asleep.

'And, actually, it only really pertains with short-term insomnia. Once insomnia becomes chronic, what matters is the third factor, the *perpetuating* factor, i.e. the gravity and momentum that keep the ball rolling. The problem is that the perpetuating factor – the activation in your brain – creates something called *conditioned arousal*, a learned response to the act of trying to fall asleep.

'So every time you start trying to fall asleep, your brain winds up and gets activated. Usually, it's because sleep has become predictably stressful. That predictable stress becomes the activation that keeps you awake. Because if, night after night, you get into bed and have trouble settling in and winding down, eventually you're going to anticipate this trouble. You'll start thinking, "Oh well, here we go again."

'So now you're climbing into bed with more activation than you had before. Which makes it harder to fall asleep. Which in turn strengthens the connection in your brain between going to bed and not being able to get to sleep. And now you're even more activated. You anticipate not sleeping, so that even if you are tired, that activation keeps you awake.

'It becomes so predictable that you don't have control over it any more. It just exists. That's why insomnia takes on a life of its own. Once you have conditioned arousal, whatever the push or kick or shove was that got the ball rolling – illness, pain, stress, whatever – becomes irrelevant, because now the only way you're going to be able to improve your sleep is to de-escalate that arousal.'

This is where CBT-I comes in: it's a protocol for retraining your brain. And it works whether you are someone who has a problem falling asleep or someone who can fall asleep quite easily to begin with, only to wake up in the middle of the night and have difficulty dropping off again.

Waking up in the night, incidentally, is subject to the same factors as being unable to fall asleep in the first place. The push – whatever it is that wakes you up, whether it's being too hot, stressed or thirsty (maybe because of snoring with your mouth open), or being disturbed by your partner snoring – causes your mind to become activated, which then gets perpetuated, and before you know it, you've created that learned response, the state of conditioned arousal, which stops you being able to go back to sleep.

The idea with CBT-I is to retrain your brain so that instead of going into conditioned arousal either at bedtime or when you find yourself awake in the middle of the night, it goes into conditioned sleepiness, so that the very act of going to bed, or of being awake in bed, is a signal to the brain to shut down – *even if it's already activated by something else.*

Dr Grandner likens it to potty training a toddler. You associate your physical interaction with a particular object – in this case, getting your body into bed – with a particular action – going to sleep.

'You're toilet training your brain,' he says. 'It's similar, because you're teaching your body to do a thing that it *can* do. That is under your control. You just don't know that it's under your control. And you can't tell yourself it's under your control. So what CBT-I does is help you shape a scaffold around the way you want it to be, to teach your brain how to do it properly. And then you remove the scaffold and it holds its shape. That's why it's like toilet training, or house training the dog. It's the same biology. In fact, it's the same learning theory. This is why it's been around for decades. It's actually not cutting-edge neuroscience. It's just good old-fashioned training.'

CBT-I technique 1: stimulus control

In stimulus control, the idea is to teach your brain that when you go to bed, only one thing happens, which is that you fall asleep. If your brain knows that getting into bed could mean any one of all sorts of other things – scrolling through social media, watching YouTube videos, doing some online shopping, watching a film, calling someone, checking emails, listening to a podcast – then you can't realistically expect it to associate getting into bed with going to sleep. The bed loses its ability to create a sleep response, the brain is activated because of stress, and then we start ruminating and overthinking, and the whole process becomes self-reinforcing.

'Instead of the bed being the sleeping place, where every once in a while other stuff happens,' Dr Grandner explains, 'the bed becomes the thinking and ruminating and not sleeping place, where occasionally sleep and other things happen. And so now the bed keeps you awake rather than puts you to sleep.'

What we have to do, he says, is take control of the *stimulus value* of the bed. You may have heard of 'learning theory', where you have a stimulus and a response, as in Pavlov's theory, in which the Pavlovian bell is the stimulus. (In Pavlov's famous experiment, dogs were conditioned to associate the ringing of the bell with the arrival of their food, so that in time, just hearing the bell was enough for them to start salivating.)

'The stimulus is the thing that you introduce into the system to get a response,' says Dr Grandner. 'Touching a hot stove is a stimulus, in that it provokes a response – pain. And, in the case of bedtime, you want getting into bed to provoke a sleep response. So you gain control, you control that stimulus value of the bed, and you reliably pair it with falling asleep. You reliably pair getting into bed with falling asleep.

'The goal is BED = SLEEP. You can't control the SLEEP side of the equation yet, but you can control the BED side of the equation. So successful stimulus control is about *not* being in bed when you're not sleeping, or when you're not going to sleep. And if you're trying to sleep and you can't sleep, then you need to not be in bed during that process.

'This alone will fix many insomnia problems for a lot of people. Of course some people say, but if I do that I may be awake all night, I may not get back to sleep at all! And I say, "Well, great. You're going to be so tired tomorrow that you'll fall asleep faster."'

CBT-I technique 2: time-restricted sleeping

The other technique – which often goes hand in hand with stimulus control – is sleep restriction therapy. The idea with this one is that you allow people to sleep a little, and once they've managed that, you allow them to sleep a little more, building up very gradually until they can sleep the whole night through.

Dr Grandner uses the analogy of a child who won't eat vegetables. You'd like them to eat 10 small pieces of broccoli but they won't even eat one. But you keep persuading them to try and eventually they manage to eat one piece. The next day you say, I know you can manage one, today let's try two. And they manage two and they say but I'm still hungry. And you say OK, can you manage three? But until they've eaten whatever that day's target is, they don't get to eat anything else. And eventually they build up to eating all 10 pieces.

Sleep restriction therapy is the same idea, says Dr Grandner, and again it's tackling the problem that your bed has become a place where you are awake, rather than a place where you are asleep.

For example, if you spend eight hours in bed but only manage to sleep for six, then six hours becomes your baseline. So instead of going to bed eight hours before you have to get up, you delay your bedtime by two hours, meaning you only have those six hours in bed in total. The question then is, can you sleep for all of those six hours?

The answer is probably not, at least at first, explains Dr Grandner. But if you stick to the process – only going to bed six hours before you have to get up – then eventually you are so tired that you do manage to sleep for the whole six hours.

'And now,' continues Dr Grandner, 'you've got a success.'

The next step is to go to bed six hours and 15 minutes before you have to get up. And if you manage to sleep for that extra 15 minutes as well, then you add another 15 minutes on to that.

'And then you wait. And then you slowly increase the time until you can't fill it any more and that's how much sleep you can regularly and reliably get.'

Studies[8] show these two techniques work as well or better than any medication, which is why, believes Dr Grandner, the American College of Physicians, the European Sleep Research Society, the Australasian Sleep Association and the US Department of Veterans' Affairs/Department of Defense all recommend that CBT-I be considered the first-line treatment for chronic insomnia.

And now you can use these techniques too. They form the central planks of the three-week reset plan for getting your sleep back on track, supplemented with many other tips and suggestions that will help support you and allow you to find exactly what works best for you and your particular needs.

HOW TO HAVE A SOOTHING BEDTIME ROUTINE

Just as children benefit from a set bedtime routine, so too do adults. Sadly, most of us don't have one, and those who don't are usually also those (one in three of us) who find it hard to fall asleep.

Matthew Walker recommends dimming the lights in your living area about an hour before you expect you'll go to bed. This has an immediate calming effect and also sends a signal to the brain to start increasing production of melatonin. He advises having very dim light in the bedroom too. Invest in plug-in nightlights, or use

---

8 Comparative effectiveness of cognitive behavioral therapy for insomnia. *BMC Family Prac.*, 2012 – link.springer.com/article/10.1186/1471-2296-13-40 and

We know CBT-1 works. Now what? *Fac. Rev.*, 2022 – doi: 10.12703/r/11-4

the torch on your phone, to avoid having to turn on bright lights if you wake in the night to go to the loo.

The important point about a bedtime routine is that it should calm you down. The idea is to have a smooth transition from your busy day to a calm night. As Dr Grandner points out, you wouldn't expect a pilot to go straight down from 37,000 feet when bringing a plane in to land; similarly, don't expect your body and brain to make a vertical descent from being highly active to extremely calm.

You'll have probably read advice about not looking at a screen before bed, but that's an unrealistic expectation for most of us. Of course, if you are disciplined enough to leave your phone and tablet or laptop in another room for the last hour before bed and indeed the rest of the night, then go right ahead.

For the less saintly among us, the important thing to remember is not to watch anything that puts you into any sort of agitated state, however mild. So it's fine to watch a favourite TV show or look at social media posts you find calming. But tense thrillers, documentaries or the news should be avoided in the last hour before bed, as should looking at X, TikTok or Insta posts that you know are likely to upset or annoy you.

Soothing yoga routines and meditation are of course excellent and highly recommended, if you enjoy them. So too is a warm bath. Our body temperature needs to drop by around 1 degree Celsius for us to fall asleep, so a warm bath seems counter-intuitive. But paradoxically, it cools us down. The warm water brings the blood to the surface, making us feel hot. That heat is then lost through our skin, bringing our core body temperature down.

One thing to avoid is a last hot drink or in fact any fluid at all in the last hour before bed. That way you are much less likely to wake up needing the loo in the middle of the night.

WHY DO WE YAWN?

Most of us think we yawn because we're tired, but sleep scientists don't think that's the main reason – many of us yawn when we're not tired, just bored, or because others are yawning. Yawning is certainly contagious – your brain is mirroring the action of someone else, which can be a very useful social and survival tool – but this is not *why* we yawn. It's now thought the main reason that we yawn is to cool down the brain.

When our brain temperature rises, we yawn more. And this, according to scientists, is so that we inhale oxygen from the outside, which is usually cooler than our core body and brain temperature and therefore cools the brain.

SNORING AND SLEEP APNOEA

We may joke about snoring, but whether you are a snorer or share a bed with one, it is a blight on a good night's sleep. Luckily, it is also one that can be remedied relatively easily.

The first thing to find out is whether your sleep position affects your snoring. If you have a partner who doesn't snore but can be relied on to be awake while you are snoring, ask them to tell you whether you snore only on your back or whether you also snore when lying on your side.

If you don't have a partner, or your partner also snores, then I suggest trying an app like Snorelab, which will record your snoring throughout the night. You can then take a few nights' recordings as a benchmark (if your partner snores you will have to sleep separately to get an accurate recording of just your own snoring level and frequency).

Once you have that benchmark, try this homemade positional device. Take a T-shirt with a front pocket. You want the T-shirt to be fairly close fitting, not loose. Then at bedtime wear it back to front and put a tennis ball in the pocket. This is an uncomfortable but effective way of stopping you sleeping on your back. Record yourself again, and if the snoring is considerably less, that's a good indicator that you need to sleep on your side. You can also buy special positional devices, and pillows, that are more comfortable (and of course more expensive) than the T-shirt/tennis ball option.

Still snoring? Try taping your mouth. Buy some microporous tape from the chemist and use it to tape over your mouth when you go to bed. This may sound a bit draconian, and it is not an attractive look, but it will force you to breathe through your nose (which is anyway much healthier). And again, if you record yourself, you will find out if mouth breathing was the cause of the snoring.

There are also exercises you can do to strengthen your throat muscles (people who sing snore much less, apparently). *Stop Snoring The Easy Way: And The Real Reasons You Need To*, by ENT consultant Dr Mike Dilkes, is an excellent and concise guide to how to do these sorts of exercises.

If you suspect your problem might be sleep apnoea rather just snoring – for example, if your partner has noticed that you sometimes stop breathing before inhaling sharply while you are asleep – you will need professional assessment. The first step is to talk to your GP, who may refer you to a sleep clinic for proper testing. You can also pay to have this done privately.

WHAT TO DO IF YOU WAKE IN THE MIDDLE OF THE NIGHT

We all wake several times during the night, usually for such brief periods that we don't even remember them. But for many people, especially those who are middle-aged or older, night-time waking can be an issue. It could be due to being too hot, perhaps because of hormonal changes – particularly in women at menopause – or needing to go to the loo, or being disturbed by some environmental factor such as noise or light. It could also be due to stress, whether that's worrying about a particular problem or just a generalised feeling of anxiety.

Whatever the cause, the first thing you will probably be tempted to do is look at the time. Resist! If you do, the next step is almost inevitable – you will start to work out how much longer before you have to get up, and then imagine how tired you'll feel if you don't get back to sleep quickly enough. That in itself is almost guaranteed to activate your brain so that indeed you won't get back to sleep quickly, because you're too busy worrying…

If sleep still seems an unlikely prospect after 30 minutes or so, get out of bed and go to another room. This is important because otherwise – just as with the conditioned arousal of associating getting into bed with insomnia described above– your brain will begin to associate being in bed with NOT sleeping.

Then, distract yourself with something calming. Avoid emails or social media and certainly don't attempt to get a jump-start on the day by doing some work – these things are guaranteed to increase your brain activation. Much better to get up and go into another room to read a book or magazine, watch a favourite TV show, draw or do something involving craftwork such as knitting, sewing, scrapbooking or even writing your thoughts in a journal.

Only go back to bed once your body and mind are calm and you feel really sleepy. You should now find you drop off quite quickly.

SELF-HYPNOSIS

My family joke that I can sleep anytime, anywhere. I maintain that's because I was exhausted for many years being a full-time working mother who took no exercise and was always desperate to sleep. But whatever the reason, it's true that I normally have no difficulty dropping off – and for decades I invariably slept straight through until morning. Then came the menopause and overpowering, drenching hot flushes that were particularly bad at night. Suddenly I was someone who most nights woke up at 3 or 4am, heart pounding, soaked in sweat.

Although the hot flushes are long gone (thank you, HRT – see the chapter on hormones for more on this and why oestrogen is vital for longevity), I still have phases of middle-of-the-night waking. Often, I go back to sleep quickly, especially when I don't look at the time. But sometimes I don't. And if I'm still awake after 20 minutes, I turn to self-hypnosis.

I learned this from Dr David Spiegel, who as Willson professor and associate chair of psychiatry & behavioral sciences, director of the Center on Stress and Health, and medical director of the Center for Integrative Medicine at Stanford University School of Medicine, is not only one of America's most lauded psychiatrists but also an expert practitioner and teacher of self-hypnosis, which he has been using as a tool to help patients for more than 40 years.

I saw him in his book-lined corner office overlooking a verdant swathe of Stanford's vast tree-lined campus, thrilled to hear in person the deep, reassuring voice that I had become accustomed to listening to in the middle of the night on his Reveri self-hypnosis app (his voice alone is probably enough to make most of us feel relaxed enough to fall back to sleep).

He launched the app out of frustration at the medical community's reluctance to embrace self-hypnosis as a tool for improving mental health, reducing anxiety and dealing with pain – despite randomised controlled trials proving it to be more effective than many drugs.

You can use self-hypnosis for almost anything – to eat better, exercise more, be less anxious, have more focus – and the app has options for all of these. But the most popular service it offers is the one for sleep. For me it works every time. See the method below if you'd like to try it, but be aware that it is probably not as good as hearing Dr Spiegel talk you through it on the app, which at the time of writing costs £89.99 a year.

Before we continue, let's just debunk the popular misconception that hypnosis is a slightly suspect trick that practitioners use to make you do strange things up on stage. In fact, it is pure science.

First, hypnosis turns down activity in two areas of the brain: the default mode network, which is the self-reflective part where you ruminate on who you are and what others think of you – the 'little ego' – and the dorsal anterior cingulate cortex, part of the salience network, which acts as an alarm system.

Secondly, it creates greater connectivity between two other brain areas: the executive control function in the prefrontal cortex and the insula, the part that helps control activities such as your breathing and heart rates.

The effect of this combination allows your body and mind to become calm, while also letting you slightly suspend your ego so that you can, as Dr Spiegel puts it, 'try on a different perspective and see what it feels like'.

'People think of hypnosis as something where somebody's controlling you, making you do things,' he adds. 'But it's actually the opposite. You are really enhancing your control over your mind and your body.

'Often when we wake up in the night we begin to get anxious. But using self-hypnosis helps both our mind and body relax within minutes. From there it's a short step to imagining ourselves in a favourite spot – say, a warm sandy beach – while we project our worries on to an imaginary screen and let them just float by. The next thing we know, it's morning and time to get up.'

LIFELINE: HOW TO USE SELF-HYPNOSIS TO GET TO SLEEP OR GET BACK TO SLEEP QUICKLY IF YOU WAKE UP IN THE NIGHT.

1. Look up to the ceiling.
2. Keeping your eyes looking up to the ceiling, close your eyelids and at the same time, inhale.
3. Keeping your eyes closed, relax them to their normal position, exhale, and imagine your body is floating.
4. Now imagine you are in a favourite place where you feel really comfortable, perhaps lying on some grass in the sun or by a mountain lake. Imagine a large screen and let your worries play out along it, just letting them go.

WHAT'S MY CHRONOTYPE?

Inside the brain is a master clock – the suprachiasmatic nucleus, a part of the hypothalamus that regulates the body's circadian system. It's responsible for the order in which certain genes are switched on and off as well as the timing of the absorption, metabolism and production of enzymes, proteins, hormones and all the other processes our bodies depend on. It's the circadian system that instructs us to be in activity mode during the day and inactivity mode at night, so it's also crucial for sleep.

The more regular our habits, from what time we eat and exercise to when we go to bed and get up, the better our bodies will function and the more precisely our circadian system can fine-tune our biological processes. But because everyone is different, no two circadian systems are exactly the same – which is why some people prefer to get up early and others late, and why some would rather do an exam mid-morning and others mid-afternoon or even early evening. This preference is determined largely by our genes, and is called our chronotype. One study[9] that looked at the Per3 circadian rhythm gene found that people with a longer allele are much more likely to be morning types, while those with a shorter allele are more likely to be evening types.

Each of us falls broadly into one of four chronotype categories:

- **Morning:** you function best if you wake up around 6am and fall asleep by 10pm.
- **Moderate morning:** you prefer to wake up around 7am and be asleep by 11pm.

---

9 A Length Polymorphism in the Circadian Clock Gene *Per3* is Linked to Delayed Sleep Phase Syndrome and Extreme Diurnal Preference. *Sleep*, 2003 – doi. org/10.1093/sleep/26.4.413

- **Moderate evening:** you prefer to wake around 7.30–8am and be asleep by midnight.
- **Evening:** you prefer to wake around 9am and be asleep by 1–2am.

(To find out which you are, here is a link for a free, five-minute quiz: https://qxmd.com/calculate/calculator_829/ morningness-eveningness-questionnaire-meq)

CAFFEINE AND ADENOSINE

Your circadian rhythm will dictate your preferences for when you wake up and when you go to bed, but there's a second force involved in what time we fall asleep. It's called sleep pressure and it's dependent on a chemical called adenosine.

Adenosine begins to build up in our brains the moment we wake up. It continues increasing throughout the day, and after around 16 hours there is so much that we begin to feel tired: our adenosine is at its peak. Assuming we then go to bed and fall asleep, one of the many things our brain does is begin to offload the adenosine. Then, next morning, if we have slept enough – i.e. 7–9 hours, depending on our individual makeup – we will wake up with the adenosine removed and our sleep pressure at its lowest point. If that happens, we wake up feeling refreshed and ready to start the day. But if we wake up still feeling tired, having not slept properly, and wishing we could have stayed in bed another hour or two, it means, among other things, that some adenosine is still present. This is why, if you wake up feeling tired, it's better to wait 90 minutes before you have your first coffee of the day, no matter how much you think you need one. Caffeine actually slows down the removal of adenosine if it's present, meaning that at night we won't feel properly sleepy at the correct time and the cycle will repeat.

HOW TO RE-ENERGISE COMPLETELY IN JUST 15 MINUTES WITH NSDR (NON-SLEEP DEEP REST, ALSO KNOWN AS YOGA NIDRA)

As I mentioned earlier, deep rest offers a wonderful and easy way to improve your health, longevity, energy and state of mind – it should be prescribed by every doctor and taught in every school.

It allows the body and brain to completely restore and rest in anything from 10 minutes to an hour. Just 30 minutes is enough to make you feel as though you've had a few hours' sleep.

It's completely free and all you need is somewhere quiet to lie down, where you won't be disturbed, and a phone or a laptop. Then you simply close your eyes and listen as someone – preferably someone with a low, calm voice that doesn't grate or jar – directs you first to take a few deep breaths, and then to turn your attention, or your focus, on to various parts of your body, in a particular sequence.

The term non-sleep deep rest was coined by Andrew Huberman, professor of neurobiology and ophthalmology at Stanford and presenter of the hugely popular podcast 'The Huberman Lab'. He explained that NSDR enhances dopamine release in one particular brain pathway – the nigrostriatal pathway – which in turn increases mental imagery and creativity. After listening to him talk about it, the CEO of Google, Sundar Pichai, tried it and now practises it regularly.

But in fact, the term NSDR is just a new name for an ancient practice that has been known to yogis for centuries – yoga nidra, or 'yoga sleep'. I have been doing yoga nidra for years and it is incredible.

You used to only be able to experience yoga nidra by going to a session at a yoga studio, but there are now many free yoga nidra sessions available on YouTube, of differing durations, and I recommend you try several to find out which you prefer. Two of my favourites are Ally Boothroyd, who has many free yoga nidras ranging from 20 minutes through to 90 minutes on YouTube, and Tim Sinesi, whose 15-minute and 10-minute yoga nidras, free on his YouTube channel Yoga With Tim, are excellent when you're short on time.

Depending on how long the session is, it might begin by asking you to focus on your right thumb, then your forefinger, middle finger, ring finger, little finger, the palm of your hand, back of your hand, wrist, forearm, right upper arm and so on through the entire right side of your body, and then the same again on the left. Or it could begin by asking you to focus on the tip of your tongue then the roof of your mouth.

It is very common to fall asleep during a session and it doesn't matter if you do, as whether you remain awake or not, your brain and body will still get exactly what they need from the practice.

At the end of the session, you will find that it takes a few minutes to slowly come back to 'normal'. When you do, you will feel calmer but also energised. Alternatively, you can use it as an aid to get to sleep – you just don't spend time coming back to your normal state and instead allow yourself to drop off.

Professor Huberman says one of the things that yoga nidra does is something most of us find very difficult, which is to switch our brain from one state to another. While most of us have no problem going from sleep to wakefulness, we find it extremely hard to switch from a state of focus to rest and back again.

Meditation achieves the same change of brain state, but Huberman, who also meditates, points out that meditation can be hard work and people often give up, whereas the beauty of yoga nidra, or NSDR, is that it is incredibly easy.

The more you do it, the more quickly you can shift your brain into a state of deep relaxation.

A number of scientific studies have shown that it is very good for your health (and therefore your longevity). In one study,[10] 20 yoga practitioners were split into two random groups. One group did conventional – hatha – yoga; the other did yoga nidra as well as hatha yoga. The findings showed that yoga nidra was much better at enhancing heart rate variability – a key indicator for longevity and health (see box on p189). Another study[11] divided participants into two groups of 60. One group did a yoga breathing technique known as nadi shodhan pranayama (alternate nostril breathing) for 30 minutes a day for four weeks; the other group did yoga nidra for 60 minutes a day for four weeks. The yoga nidra group showed significantly greater reductions in blood pressure, pulse rate, breath rate and body mass index, as well as reductions in anxiety.

And another four-year study of 41 chronic insomnia sufferers[12] found that yoga nidra reduced cortisol significantly and also improved stages 2 and 3 of sleep, as well as overall sleep quality.

---

10 Yoga Nidra Relaxation Increases Heart Rate Variability and is Unaffected by a Prior Bout of Hatha Yoga. *J. Alt. and Comp. Med.*, 2012 – doi.org/10.1089/acm.2011.0331

11 A comparative study of Yoga Nidra and Nadisodhana Pranayam on essential hypertension. *Adv Sci Lett.* 2016 – doi: 10.1166/asl.2016.6834

12 Yoga Nidra practice shows improvement in sleep in patients with chronic insomnia. *Natl. Med. J. India*, 2021 – 34(3):143–150. 10.25259/NMJI_63_19. [DOI] [PubMed]

RESTING MORE DEEPLY:
The three-week reset

WEEK 1: making changes
SUNDAY

Start your sleep diary today. Make a note of the following:

- What time you woke up.
- How rested you felt when you woke up: Really good, ready to start the day?/OK, but wish I could have slept longer?/Not great – really don't feel rested?/Terrible – feel exhausted?
- Your physical state: Clear eyes, not dehydrated, plenty of energy?/Dry mouth? Headache? Too hot?
- Whether you woke up in the night and if so, why: I needed to go to the loo/I was too hot/too cold/I was thirsty/I had a bad dream/I was in an uncomfortable position in bed/A noise woke me/My partner was snoring/I was snoring (it is worth trying to remedy this – see p162).
- How long it took you to get back to sleep. And if you couldn't go back to sleep for 30 minutes or longer, why was that? For example, I was worried about something going on in my life right now/I was worried about the day ahead/I was worried that I couldn't get back to sleep and how tired I would be the next day.

Then, just before you are ready to go to bed, make a note of the following:

- What time you had your last cup of coffee.
- What you ate in the evening and when.
- What you had to drink, and when.
- What you did in the evening before bed – for example, watched a film or TV series, played video games, looked at social media, did household chores.
- What time it was when you decided to go to bed, and how sleepy you felt.

Now for three critical changes to your sleep routine.

1. Don't go to bed until you feel sleepy. Dr Michael Grandner likens this to not forcing yourself to eat if you're not hungry. Just as it makes no sense to sit down at the dining table waiting to get hungry, so it is pointless to lie in bed waiting to feel sleepy. All you will do is make yourself stressed.

   So, if you don't feel sleepy – hold off going to bed. Do something distracting but peaceful, such as reading a book or listening to a podcast. Don't work, or watch a film, or scroll through social media. Activities like these are known by sleep scientists as arousal activities – and they don't mean it in a good way. They make your mind too active for sleep.

   It doesn't matter how long that takes; you may end up going to bed two or three hours later than you would do normally. The point is, if you only get into bed when you are actually ready to sleep, you are much more likely to fall asleep and stay asleep. And don't worry if that means you are getting less sleep than you think you need. A few (or even many) nights of less than the ideal amount of sleep really won't matter in the long run. They are not going to give you dementia or impair your brain function. They are just a blip on the way to getting your sleep right.

2. Get up at your normal time, no matter how late it was when you went to sleep. Maybe you have to be up for work in the morning, or to get the children ready for school, or to meet someone, or go to an exercise class, or let the plumber in. Perhaps you have no commitments at all. It doesn't matter: stick to the time you normally get up, *no matter what*.

3. If you are someone who regularly wakes up in the middle of the night, and, after trying for 25–30 minutes, you haven't managed to get back to sleep, get up. Go to another room and do something calming. Tempting though it might be to get a jump-start on the week ahead, definitely don't do anything connected to work (unless it's to make a plan that will help you with something and therefore make you feel calmer). If you are anxious, you could write down your thoughts, which may also be calming. What you are aiming to do is distract yourself from the anxiety of not being able to get back to sleep, and from any spiralling thoughts about how tired you're now going to be in the morning and how that's going to impact your day. Read a book, do some crafting, or watch something gentle and unchallenging. Do not get back into bed until, or unless, you feel really sleepy.

MONDAY

As you did on Sunday, make a note in your sleep diary of what time you woke up, how you feel, whether you woke up in the night and why. If snoring is an issue, note what remedy, if any, you tried and whether it made any difference.

Then as soon as you can, go outside. Getting as much natural daylight as possible after waking sends a very clear signal to your brain that now it is morning, so the pineal gland can stop releasing melatonin. This is very important. Not only does it understand that the day has begun; it also understands that the evening will begin approximately 12 hours from now – when it will start releasing melatonin again. This in turn ensures that we begin to feel sleepy and ready for sleep a few hours after that.

You can use this time outside to be physically active – to go for a walk, or do some exercise or gardening – or you can simply sit, and perhaps use it as an opportunity for meditation or breathwork (for more on these, go to page 187). If you have long enough, you can do both. The ideal time to spend outside first thing is 30–45 minutes – but even a few minutes are better than none, so do whatever you can. Make a note in your sleep diary.

If you are a coffee drinker – which I am, devotedly – then bear in mind that as it takes caffeine 8–10 hours to leave your system, it will almost certainly interfere with your body's natural sleep rhythm unless you are careful about what time you drink it. Decide what time you want to go to sleep this evening and subtract 10 hours from that time as the cut-off point for your last cup of coffee. (for example, I want to go to sleep at 11pm, so I need to remember not to drink coffee after 1pm.)

Evening: again, make a note of what time you get into bed, what you did this evening and what you had to eat and drink. As before, only get into bed when you feel very sleepy, even if that means going to bed one, two or even three hours later than usual. And make sure you get up at the same time tomorrow as you did today – no matter what.

TUESDAY

Morning: fill in your sleep diary when you wake up, and then go outside as soon as you can.

Decide what time you would like to be asleep by and make a mental note of the latest time you can finish drinking coffee.

Evening: continue with whatever snoring remedy you have chosen – it takes a while to get used to sleeping on your side, or sleeping with your mouth taped, so persevere, because not snoring will make a huge difference to your quality of sleep. Not only will you wake up feeling more rested, but you will also be much less dehydrated and therefore less likely to have a headache.

Again, make a note of what time you get into bed, what you did this evening and so on. And make sure you get up at the same time tomorrow as you did today – no matter what.

WEDNESDAY

Morning: fill in your sleep diary, and go outside.

Today, in addition to thinking about what time you have your coffee, we're also going to think about when you have your last drink of the day. For example, if your last drink is a large glass of water or a large mug of camomile tea half an hour before getting into bed, you are placing quite a burden on your bladder for the next seven or eight hours. If you are waking regularly in the middle of the night to go to the loo, this may well be why. So today, have your last drink of the evening at least an hour but preferably *90 minutes to two hours* before bed. Then have just a very small glass of water by your bed so that you don't worry about being thirsty in the night or when you wake up.

Only go to bed when you feel properly sleepy, set your alarm for the same time as on the previous days – and get up at that time, no matter how tired you might feel.

THURSDAY

Do as for Wednesday, but with one addition. Today you are going to look carefully at what you are doing in the hour or two before bed and think about introducing a soothing bedtime routine.

As Dr Grandner says, you can't make a vertical descent from 37,000 feet and expect everything to go smoothly. It's the same with sleep. If you spend the hour before you go to bed watching a tense thriller or a documentary about a serial killer, or playing a demanding video game, or being incensed by something you've seen on X or TikTok, or upset by something horrible on the news, then it is highly unlikely you will fall asleep easily when you do get into bed. Your mind is too agitated.

He points out that we make sure children have a regular, soothing routine before bedtime – and we should do the same. It is unrealistic, he thinks, for people to stop looking at their screens completely. But as a guide, if whatever you are looking at – a film, a game, social media – is so immersive that you can't bear to drag yourself away, you will find it very difficult to switch off and drift off to sleep when you get into bed. Choose instead to do those activities much earlier in the evening and make it a rule to finish at least one hour, preferably two, before you want to go to sleep.

As an alternative to activities that put you into an agitated state before sleep, think about what a soothing routine would look like for you, and experiment with one this evening. Perhaps a warm bath or some restorative yoga, or maybe just watching something you are familiar with and find comforting, rather than addictive or thrilling. Plan your evening so that you can begin that routine in good time before bed.

FRIDAY

As for Thursday. And, even though tomorrow is Saturday, do your best to stick to the same times for going to bed and waking up. If you enjoyed your evening routine from yesterday, do it again tonight. If not, experiment with something else. It really doesn't matter what it is, as long as you find it soothing.

SATURDAY

By now you may be starting to have a feel for what particular pitfalls sleep holds for you and what elements of the new routine are beginning to help. We will be looking at this in detail next week. But for now, continue with everything you've been doing all week. If you are going out – it is Saturday, after all! – and can't go to bed at the same time, then just accept that. This is real life. But to give yourself the best chance of success, make a choice during these three weeks to keep late nights to a minimum and prioritise your sleep routine.

WEEK 2: troubleshooting
SUNDAY

Hopefully you are now starting to form a habit of filling in your sleep diary as soon as you can after waking up, then going outside, and knowing what time your last coffee of the day should be.

Take some time today to look over last week's diary. Do any patterns emerge? For example, what would you identify as your main sleep problem? Is it that you have trouble falling asleep? Difficulty going back to sleep after waking in the night? Waking up too early and not being able to go back to sleep? Falling asleep OK and staying asleep OK but nevertheless waking up feeling tired and headachy? Or is there some other factor in play?

Next, identify how frequent the problem is. Every night? Most nights? Three or four nights?

Then have a look at why you think the problem is happening. Could it be connected to caffeine still in your system? Mind-activating films, games or social media too close to bedtime? Snoring? Needing the loo? An uncomfortable bed or pillow? The external environment?

On the nights when you slept better, can you work out why?

Next, try to work out how you feel about any interventions you made. For example, you may feel frustrated that despite going to bed only when you felt sleepy, and waking up at the same time no matter what, there hasn't been much of an improvement.

Consider the pros and cons attached to that. A pro could be that at least you have more of a feeling of being in control, of taking charge of the problem. A con could be that you feel like giving up and that it's not working; maybe despite having given up your habitual mid-afternoon coffee, the problem hasn't resolved. A pro could be that although change is difficult, you've done it – and the fact that the problem hasn't yet resolved doesn't necessarily prove that mid-afternoon coffee is not the cause. It may be a contributing factor, alongside some other thing you have yet to discover.

Make a list of interventions and identify as many pros and cons as you can. Then go through each one, deciding: do I keep this intervention or ditch it? Before you ditch it, though, remember that this was only week 1! You got through it – and there are only two more weeks to go. As time goes by, not only will the changes become easier and more habitual, but your sleep *will* improve.

To be clear: this three-week plan is only a reset. But it is strongly evidence-based and will put you very firmly on the path for long-term, positive sleep success. Realistically, if you have deeply ingrained sleep behaviours that need changing, it will be between six and eight weeks before you see major success. The good news is that, when your sleep does start improving, it will just keep getting better – and the change will be lasting. A recent study by Dr Grandner's team found that, even two years after attending their sleep clinic, patients' sleep continued to improve, with them sleeping on average 45 minutes longer than after they'd been successfully treated.

For week 2, there are some more changes to make, to do with light and temperature. You will sleep much more deeply in a room that is dark and cool. If you can, invest in blackout blinds or curtains. If that's too much right now, buy a sleep mask to block out unwanted light (and ear plugs, too, if noise is an issue).

Next, turn the radiator in your bedroom right down (or even off altogether). In order to fall asleep, the body's temperature needs to drop by just under 1 degree Celsius (2–3 Fahrenheit); it will then rise by a few degrees when it's time to wake up. So it makes sense to keep your room as cool as possible. Professor Matthew Walker says the ideal temperature is 16.5C or 67F. If that feels too cold, don't make the room warmer. It's better to instead change your bedding, for example, from one thick duvet to layers: perhaps a sheet, topped by a thinner duvet, and one or two blankets that you can throw off as necessary. If you and your partner fundamentally disagree on what is cool and what is warm, the answer is simple: have a (smaller) duvet each! (Paradoxically, a warm bath can help us sleep – see p161).

This week it would be good to also think about dimming the lights in your living area an hour or so before bed. You'll be surprised at how sleepy this makes you feel. It's to do with melatonin: just as getting sunlight first thing tells the body to stop releasing it, so dimming the lights in the evening gives the signal to start releasing it again. Make sure the light in your bedroom is dim too. If you want to read, use a targeted reading lamp with a narrow, focused concentration of light. Another good idea is to install plug-in night lights to light the way to the bathroom. Once there, use the torch on your phone or another nightlight rather than flood your brain with bright light.

And finally, use this week to experiment with cutting down on evening alcohol, which contrary to a common misconception, doesn't help with sleep at all. As Professor Walker says: 'You may fall asleep easily and feel like you stay asleep, but there are three issues. The first is that alcohol is in a class of drugs called sedatives – and sedation is not sleep. The second is that because it's sedation, the electrical signature of your deep sleep is not the same – there are components no longer present when you have alcohol in your system, and others that are abnormally present. Alcohol also fragments your sleep with awakenings throughout the night. You don't remember because they're brief. But you wake up not feeling restored.

'The final concern is that it's quite a potent blocker of REM sleep [when we dream] and so you lose out on the incredible memory, creativity and emotional regulation benefits that come with that.'

MONDAY

Fill in your sleep diary and then continue with interventions: go outside as early as you can; think carefully about when to have coffee, and also alcohol; check that your bedroom is cool and dark; disengage from anything that overexcites or agitates your mind for at least an hour before bed; dim the lights in your living area an hour before bed, and keep the bedroom light dim too.

This week it is time to start looking more closely at the amount of sleep you are actually getting.

For example: if you discover that, as a result of delaying going to bed until you were definitely sleepy last week, you are getting an average of six hours' sleep, you can now experiment and see if you can expand that time a little. Try going to bed 15 minutes earlier.

TUESDAY

As for Monday, including – if you managed to fall asleep relatively quickly – going to bed 15 minutes earlier.

Today you could also experiment with using self-hypnosis as a tool for getting back to sleep, or settling down before sleep. Try Dr David Spiegel's app, Reveri, which will guide you through a short but astonishingly effective self-hypnosis session to help you fall asleep or get back to sleep if you wake in the night (see box on p167).

WEDNESDAY

As for Tuesday, but if you have been delaying going to bed for an hour or more until you feel sleepy and you have found that going to bed 15 minutes earlier has worked on Monday and/or Tuesday, try today bringing your bedtime forward by a further 15 minutes. The idea is that you gradually bring your bedtime back to where you would like it to be, but incrementally in steps.

Continue with all other interventions.

THURSDAY and FRIDAY

Continue with all interventions. If you are waking in the middle of the night, continue with self-hypnosis and/or going into another room, only getting back into bed when you feel really sleepy. And, of course, keep filling in your sleep diary.

SATURDAY

Continue with all interventions. If at all possible, try to avoid a late night, just for the next few weeks.

Week 3: honing your sleep plan so that it is perfect for YOU

Set aside some time at the beginning of this week to go through last week's sleep diary, looking for what has worked, and what hasn't. On average, would you say you are sleeping better than you were before you started this plan? If the answer is no, explore why – did you abandon interventions too soon? What did you find difficult? Can you think of a way to make things easier? Perhaps you don't after all really need or want to sleep better than you already do?

If you are sleeping better, make a note of what seems to be working – lighting? Temperature? Stopping snoring? Sleep restriction (i.e., not getting into bed until really sleepy)? Not napping? Caffeine timing? Alcohol intake?

If waking in the middle of the night was your biggest problem, how has that changed? Do you still wake but get back to sleep more quickly? If so, why is that? Is it simply because you now drink less fluid before going to bed? Did cutting back on alcohol make a difference? Did self-hypnosis help? Did you manage to avoid looking at the time? Which distraction activities did you find best?

It is also useful to note whether the frequency of your sleep difficulties has changed. How many nights did you have problems this week compared to last? And most important of all – how has the quality of your sleep changed?

Armed with details, you can now set about tailoring your sleep plan to your precise needs.

If you think, having tried it, that there is an intervention that doesn't really help, then stop doing it this week and see if it makes any difference. Conversely, identify those interventions that seem to work particularly well for you, and prioritise them above all else.

For Bryan Johnson, those are:

1. Prioritise your bedtime – it's the most important appointment of your day.
2. Read or listen to a book for 15 minutes before bed.
3. Tell yourself it's time to go to sleep.
4. Redirect any anxieties or ideas or thoughts on your to-do list to tomorrow, when you will have all day.
5. No screens.
6. Don't eat late.
7. Have a 30-minute wind-down before bed.
8. Don't take stimulants late in the day.
9. Keep your bedroom temperature neither too hot nor too cold.
10. Find the sleep position that works for you.

Given that he says he sleeps perfectly – on average eight and a half hours – almost every night, I think it's important to share his advice.

So this week, keep your sleep diary and continue with all interventions that have worked for you. If gradually bringing your bedtime forward is working, then advance it by 15 minutes today, Monday and Tuesday, and by another 15 minutes, if appropriate, on Wednesday, Thursday, Friday and Saturday. That makes an hour earlier in total. Continue bringing your bedtime forward in the weeks to come if necessary, until you have reached a time that allows you to fall asleep quickly – within 10 or 15 minutes of deciding it's time to sleep – and also get the optimum amount of sleep for you (for most of us, that's between seven and eight hours).

5
STRESS, HAPPINESS
& HOW TO MAKE
A HABIT STICK

Stress, as I mentioned right at the beginning of this book, is one of the greatest obstacles to longevity. When we are stressed, everything becomes secondary to simply surviving the enormous burden of tension and strain we carry. It is difficult to eat properly, or exercise or sleep. And it creates a vicious cycle – the less we do those things, the more stressed we become. Carry on like this and, sooner or later, something will break.

This is why I suggested earlier that Deepak Chopra's single tip for a better life – take it easy, disengage from the drama – is probably worth the cost of his Life and Longevity retreat on its own. And my advice to you is to find one thing – just one thing – that helps you let go.

When I say one thing, I don't mean drink or drugs, which of course will only make things a whole lot worse. Do whatever it takes to find something else.

Here is a more radical suggestion. Just before you brush your teeth in the morning, look at yourself in the mirror and say – *out loud*: 'Life is for me. I love life. I deserve fun. I deserve happiness.

I deserve time to relax. I relax into the flow of life and release control. Life is a joy, and life is for me.'

Unless you are extremely open-minded, you will find this almost impossible. It will make you feel silly. You will tell yourself it's a ridiculous suggestion and that you are not an idiot. All I ask is that you try it. It is free. No one needs to know. And it works.

So, if you are stressed (and who isn't?), for the next three weeks say these few words as many times a day as possible, whenever you have a spare 30 seconds.

Say them when you're going to work. Say them when you're walking to a meeting. Say them when you're queuing to pay. Say them when you're waiting for the kettle to boil. Say them when you're stuck in a traffic jam. Say them while you're getting ready for bed, or about to fall asleep. Just keep saying them – and I guarantee your stress will start to lessen.

THE 10-SECOND OR COHERENT BREATH

This is one of the best ways I know to reduce stress and anxiety, to calm and clear your mind. Find somewhere quiet and comfortable to sit on a straight-backed chair. It can be helpful to put a small cushion behind you at the base of your spine, so that your lower back is supported. Keep your spine straight, shoulders down and relaxed, feet flat on the floor. Think about relaxing your jaw – we often carry a lot of tension here without realising it. Start by simply noticing your breath – not trying to change it in any way, just noticing it. Then take a deep inhale through your nose, and exhale through your mouth. And then again. Hopefully by now you are feeling calm and relaxed.

Now it is time to begin the 10-second, or coherent, breath. It can be helpful to place one hand on your stomach for this. Inhale through your nose to a slow count of four and, as you do, consciously think about your stomach expanding so that you feel a gentle movement under your hand. Then exhale through your nose to a slow count of four, and feel your stomach muscles gently contract so that your hand slightly moves down. You will notice a slight pause after each inhale and exhale – that's fine, and what you want.

The idea is to breathe like this for around 10 minutes, and to practise it every day.

For some, this breathwork will feel completely natural; others, though, will find it extremely hard. If it's impossible for you at first to make either your inhale or exhale last to a slow count to four, then reduce it to three. As you do it more, you will find you can increase the duration of each inhale and exhale. We typically breathe 10–20 times a minute, and the more stressed we are, the more quickly and shallowly we breathe. We're aiming, with this exercise, to slow our breathing down to 6–10 breaths per minute – this may take you some time to get right.

Many studies[1] have shown that breathing in this way changes the pattern of signals in the brain, allowing brain waves to synchronise across larger areas. By slowing our breathing down, we also slow our heartbeat and activate our calming, parasympathetic nervous system. In addition, it enhances heart rate variability (HRV) – the higher your HRV, the greater your longevity (see box opposite).

At the end of 10 minutes of this coherent breathing, you may feel simultaneously calm and yet more alert. If you are extremely

---

1 The physiological effects of slow breathing in the healthy human. Breathe, 2017 – breathe.ersjournals.com/content/13/4/298

stressed, though, it may take a while for you to feel the full effects. Just trust in the process. You will be amazed by how much better you start to feel if you practise every day.

This sort of breathing has been practised for thousands of years, in both Chinese medicine and Indian yoga. In fact, yoga was originally more focused on breath control than physical postures.

What is heart rate variability?

HRV is the variability in the rate at which our heart beats based on the needs of our body and respiratory patterns. Our heartbeat needs to be flexible, in order to be able to change depending on what we're doing – to go faster when we're exercising hard or when we're stressed, and slower when we're calm and relaxed. And our HRV is a measure of how adaptable our body is. A highly variable heart rate is generally a sign of cardiovascular fitness and resilience, while a low HRV shows our body is less resilient and struggles to adapt to change and can be an augur of current or future health problems. HRV decreases quite sharply with age, so while the average 30-year-old is likely to have an HRV in the 50–85 range, 60–65-year-olds tend to be in the 25–45 range.

It's difficult to measure accurately without specialised equipment, although there are various wearable devices you can buy that claim to measure it, including Apple watches and Whoop.

CYCLIC SIGHING – AND SINGING

Many of us think that we're driven to breathe in air because we need more oxygen. In fact, it's not low oxygen that drives the need to inhale, but high carbon dioxide. The body is even more sensitive to high carbon dioxide than it is to low oxygen and so we inhale in order to immediately exhale the excess CO_2. But if we breathe too quickly, we are actually exhaling too much carbon dioxide, which affects the balance between the two in the blood.

This can lead to a feeling of panic. In a panic attack, a person may genuinely fear they are suffocating and can't breathe, but they will, in fact, have plenty of oxygen in their blood. What happens is that the 'fight or flight' response, or the sympathetic nervous system, is triggered, and the blood then gets suffused with oxygen – which, if we were genuinely facing a threat where we needed to fight or run, would be used up and burned off. However, if we are not running or physically active, the oxygen in our blood remains high and the carbon dioxide too low. This is why it helps to breathe into a paper bag – that way we breathe back in the carbon dioxide we've exhaled into it, allowing the balance to restore itself in the blood.

Most of us breathe too quickly. But a remarkable study by David Spiegel and Professor Andrew Huberman found that just five minutes a day of cyclic sighing – where you do two quick inhales, followed by a long exhale – is not only immediately calming, but also lowers people's average respiratory rate over an entire 24-hour period.

Try it. You will feel your body instantly starting to relax.

Dr Spiegel believes it also increases HRV.

'Five minutes once a day is plenty,' he says. He also points out that we are programmed to sigh periodically. One example is when we are sad. A sigh can convey a sort of emotional acceptance. Gratifyingly, singing has a similar effect as it involves a quick inhale then a longer exhale, and it is one reason why Dr Spiegel believes singing is such a favourite human activity. It's not just about the music, or the fact that it is communal; it genuinely calms us down and makes us feel better.

MINDFULNESS AND MEDITATION

There are countless studies showing the benefits of mindfulness and meditation, which are really one and the same thing.

In mindfulness, you typically concentrate on counting the breath in order to stay focused on the present moment (for example, mentally say 1 as you inhale, 2 as you exhale, 3 as you inhale, 4 as you exhale – up to 10, and then begin again). But it doesn't have to be the breath – you could focus on a particular sound, or activity, like walking.

In meditation, you may also simply count the breath. But you can also focus on repeating a sound, or mantra, over and over again in your head. Many people find this kind of meditation – known as deep, or transcendental, meditation – very easy to do. But because it can take you very deep it needs to be done – initially at least – under the guidance of a properly qualified and experienced meditation teacher.

Like coherent breathing and cyclic sighing, it slows your respiratory rate down, bringing numerous health benefits.

What both mindfulness and meditation allow you to do is connect with yourself more and in the process be more content with what you have and where you are right now. It helps you feel calmer and, crucially, more aware. Being present in the moment, rather than letting your mind leap forwards and backwards, means you can concentrate more on what is happening right now – so that you focus completely on the person you're listening to, or the piece of work you're doing, or the run you're on. As a result, you'll find you connect more with the person, complete the work better and find the run easier and more enjoyable. Equally, it will help you stay calm in a stressful situation, whether that's sitting in a traffic jam or dealing with bad news.

Studies show that just three minutes of meditation a day brings benefits. However you choose to do it, you will find you have improved focus. And being in the present moment is one of the best ways to boost happiness. Instead of focusing on what has happened, or worrying about what might happen, you are focusing on being right here, right now.

A common misconception is that this means you have to stop thinking. That's not the point at all. The point is that you are focusing on just one thing – be that your breath, or a sound or walking. We can't stop our thoughts, because our minds are designed to think. But for the period of mindfulness or meditation we are engaged in, we can choose not to focus on them – to just acknowledge they are there, and then let them drift past.

This doesn't mean you won't get distracted. Despite your best efforts, your attention will wander away from time to time and pursue a thought. But simply realising that your attention has wandered is enough to enable you to note it and let it pass, then come back again to your breath or whatever your focus is. It doesn't matter how many times this happens, as long as you bring your attention back each time. So, think of the practice of mindfulness and meditation as a practice of refocusing. That's where the magic happens.

There are various subscription-based apps that you can use – Waking Up and Headspace are both good places to start. There are also many free meditations on YouTube. My favourite meditations are with Eckhart Tolle, also free.

HOW TO BE HAPPY

The answer is actually much simpler than you might think. And anyone who has ever watched the brilliant survival TV series *Alone* will know the answer.

In *Alone*, for those who haven't seen it, 10 survival experts – Bear Grylls types who can knock up a sturdy shelter in the middle of nowhere with nothing but a bit of timber and some leaves, who can start a fire with two sticks and aren't remotely fazed by the fact that it's freezing and there's not a supermarket or coffee shop within 300 miles – are sent to the wilderness that is Vancouver Island and left to fend for themselves. (Yes, confusing for us Brits, who tend to think of Vancouver Island as the first of many luxury havens that Harry and Meghan relocated to after deciding that the royal life of duty, combined with having to live in draughty country houses with no mixer taps, was not for them).

The *Alone* participants are only allowed to bring 10 items with them; in addition, they are each given a satellite phone that they can use to send a distress signal if they decide they have had enough and want to leave. The winner is the last man or woman left standing. Because they are completely alone, they film themselves, so there are no cameramen. And obviously, none of the participants know who might have left, or how many are still in the game. They only know they've won when the boat arrives to tell them so.

So why do you think they leave? Is it because they are starving, scared and cold? The answer is no. What tends to happen is that they manage to build themselves wonderful shelters, devise extraordinary ways of catching food, build spectacular fires and in some cases boats, tables and chairs. Along the way they deal with various extreme annoyances – grizzly bears, let's say, or semi-starvation – but, generally, after six weeks or so they are surviving rather beautifully (one man even found a long, hollow stick that he was able to utilise as a urinal so that he didn't even have to leave his shelter in the middle of the night to pee).

The reason they leave is not the discomfort, the fear or the hunger, although they are constantly battling these issues. The reason is loneliness. In the end, even these people – resilient, resourceful, courageous, optimistic, good-humoured, extraordinary human beings most of us would be completely humbled by – leave because they just can't stand being on their own.

Which brings me to Harvard, and an 85-year study that set out to find out what makes us happy in life. Answer: other people. Social connections.

Robert Waldinger, who directs that study and is a professor of psychiatry at Harvard, says that when it comes to our relationships, we need seven keystones of support:

1. **Safety and security:** Who would you call if you woke up scared in the middle of the night? Who would you turn to in a moment of crisis?
2. **Learning and growth:** Who encourages you to try new things, to take chances, to pursue your life's goals?
3. **Emotional closeness and confiding:** Who knows everything (or most things) about you? Who can you call on when you're feeling low and be honest with about how you're feeling?

4. **Identity affirmation and shared experience:** Is there someone in your life who has shared many experiences with you and who helps you strengthen your sense of who you are?
5. **Romantic intimacy:** Do you feel satisfied with the amount of romantic intimacy in your life?
6. **Help (both informational and practical):** The person you turn to if you need some expertise or help solving a practical problem (e.g., planting a tree, fixing your WiFi connection).
7. **Fun and relaxation:** Who makes you laugh? Who do you call to see a movie or go on a road trip with? Who makes you feel connected and at ease?

We need different people to fulfil these roles, and not all the roles might matter to us. But Professor Waldinger says that going through the list and identifying any gaps that there may be in our life is a way of 'seeing below the surface of our social universe'. Either way, for a long and healthy life, it's not enough to be physically and mentally fit. We need a high level of social fitness too.

WE *ARE* OUR HABITS

It may sound counter-intuitive but the process of habit-building is in some ways the very essence of mindfulness. One of the key things I've learned from mindfulness is that all we have is the present moment. It sounds obvious but it's not how we tend to view life.

We get caught in thinking obsessively about what has happened, or what might happen. We get so wrapped up in thinking about the past and the future that we completely forget about now.

And yet *now is the only place that change can happen* – not in the past, and not at some future moment that hasn't yet arrived.

This is important to remember when it comes to changing habits. To a great extent, we *are* our habits. Whether we've intended to develop them or not, they are part of our everyday lives and therefore part of who we are.

So changing even just three habits is not going to be easy. However, that very act of trying to change, that moment-to-moment effort, is not only part of the process of change – it *is* the change.

If, when I started out on my health journey, my goal had been to knock four decades off my biological age, then I would almost certainly have failed. I would have found the idea utterly ridiculous.

What actually happened was that my goal at the beginning was just to fix my back. I knew I needed a stronger core to do that, and so that's what I focused on, by going to Pilates classes.

I'd never done Pilates (or indeed any regular exercise) and can still remember how agonisingly sore my muscles were the next day. But I went back a couple of days later because I had a very clear memory of being almost unable to walk for a few weeks after injuring my back. I realised this was how it must feel to be very old and I really didn't want to feel like that ever again.

So, although I found it hard going, I made myself keep at it. I had to force myself to go to the classes. And then, after a while, I realised I was starting to look forward to them. Apart from anything else, I was so intently focused on getting through each exercise that there was no room in my head to think about anything else – and it dawned on me how restorative that was mentally.

It wasn't long before I began to feel the physical effects too. Very gradually my body shape began to change, until one day I looked in the mirror and realised I had some muscle definition in my legs and arms. My goal changed from wanting not just to fix my back, but to getting my entire body fitter and stronger.

Suddenly I was going to Pilates three or four times a week and *enjoying* it, relishing my progress from beginner to intermediate, using heavier weights and resistance and seeing my body shape become more and more defined. The stronger I started to feel, the stronger I looked, which in turn made me feel even stronger. It was a virtuous circle.

After a year or two of Pilates, I felt brave enough to try Bikram yoga, as there happened to be a studio near where I lived. I'd done it once, years before, with a friend and had been so bamboozled by the intensity of it that I immediately googled afterwards 'has anyone ever died doing Bikram yoga?'

Now I found that I loved it. I wasn't very flexible but I was certainly stronger. So now I was going to Pilates three times a week and Bikram yoga two or three times a week. Without even meaning to, in the space of just 18 months, I'd formed an impressive exercise habit, going from almost zero to six days a week.

I believe the key to it was that, yes, I was motivated, but at the same time it happened *gradually*. Aged 47, I really didn't want to feel like an old lady who struggled to walk. But I didn't, on day one, decide I had to go from almost never exercising to doing it six days a week. If I had done that, I would certainly have failed.

Instead, I did it bit by bit – and you can too.

Don't think you can master the three habits I have outlined in this book in a few weeks and then crack the longevity problem. You can't, and you won't. What you can do is start improving your longevity chances, little by little, day by day. Remember, it's not time that turns an action into a habit, but frequency – i.e. it's not how *long* you spend doing it, but how *often* you do it. The more often you do something, the more quickly it will become automatic.

Start small. The change is not what happens when you reach the end of a particular goal. The change is happening because of what you're doing right now, step by step, moment by moment.

In his book *Atomic Habits*, which I highly recommend, James Clear suggests the 'Two Minute Rule', whereby you begin forming a new habit by breaking it down to just two minutes. So, for example, if you want to start walking every day, walk for two minutes – then stop. If you want to start going regularly to the gym, go there – but after two or five minutes, leave. (He had one client whose goal was to lose weight. After a few weeks of regularly going to the gym for just five minutes, one day he thought: 'Well, since I come here all the time anyway, I may as well spend a bit longer.' He lost more than five stone.)

You may feel like this is a way of tricking yourself (a bit like retraining your brain by depriving yourself of sleep in order to ensure that when you do go to bed you associate that place with being asleep – see p157), but if it achieves the goal of doing your new habit frequently, all well and good. *Any* time spent exercising or eating more healthily is better for the goal of living a longer, healthier life than no time spent at all.

EASY DOES IT

Above all, you need to make doing your new habit as easy as possible and make sure you reward yourself regularly along the way with healthy but enjoyable pleasures such as a massage or a bubble bath.

If you can see the process of working towards your goal as a series of enjoyable experiences, you will be able to release the stress and worry of not achieving it.

One small change will lead to another, which in time will lead to another and then another. Suddenly, you will find that a series of tiny changes has grown to a significant change, almost without your realising.

Don't be discouraged if you forget to practise your habit after a few days or backslide. A journey of a thousand miles begins with a single step – but along the way you won't always be putting one foot in front of the other and making steady progress; sometimes you will hit a bump in the road that forces you to divert or stop.

That doesn't matter, as long as you keep your destination in mind and resume the journey as soon as you can.

HOW TO STAY MOTIVATED

Something else that will help keep you on track is a small exercise recommended by Middlesex University's Dr Rhonda Cohen, a sport and exercise psychologist. She explains that motivation can be either 'intrinsic', meaning we do it for ourselves, or 'extrinsic', meaning we do it for external reasons – for instance, the 'reward' of knowing that our family will benefit from knowing we will be around for a long time. 'With intrinsic motivation for longevity, for example, we are self-challenged; we want to master the skills or routines we need so we can enjoy a healthy long life,' she explains. 'With extrinsic motivation, we are more challenged by the idea of accomplishing a task for an external reward.'

She suggests you first decide what motivational type you are, and then look at what you need to progress. 'If you're intrinsically motivated then ask yourself what you are looking to gain with each step, and decide how to celebrate each achievement. If you're more externally motivated, then what rewards will you give yourself when you reach your goals – for example, will you buy yourself some new clothes for exercising?' (And of course you may be a bit of both, in which case you can alternate the types of rewards.)

Beware critical thinking too. 'If you know you have a tendency to compare yourself to others, then work on the idea of your personal best. Don't blame yourself if you are not perfect – who is? Keep trying, as this is your life's show! And don't use an "all or nothing" approach either. Remember things aren't always one way or the other. There's always an inbetween.'

Bad day?

We all have low points – being rejected by someone, not achieving the result we wanted, feeling low. That's when we reach for the junk food. Trust me, even after years of diligent exercise and healthy eating, there are days when I can't be bothered to go to the gym or for a run, when I reach for the millionaire's shortbread or pepperoni pizza – or both.

Here's my rescue remedy to get yourself back on track:

1. Forgive yourself.
2. Have a luxurious bath, or better still treat yourself to a massage.
3. Give yourself a stern talking-to: today is allowed; tomorrow is not.
4. Plan your exercise and your food for tomorrow – the what, where, when, how.
5. Go to bed early so you can wake up feeling refreshed and ready to pick things up again.

6

HORMONES, VITAMINS & SUPPLEMENTS

Suppose I told you that there was a miracle supplement you could take that would increase your lifespan by 40 years, while also restoring your energy levels to those of someone half your age.

Sounds tempting, doesn't it? And it's backed up by impressive research. But there's a snag: at the moment, the bulk of that research is only in mice.

That hasn't stopped people from racing to take it, though. The miracle supplement is NMN – nicotinamide mononucleotide (for more on this, see p211) – and it's just one example of the confusing and expensive world of longevity supplementation and anti-ageing products.

The longevity game is big, big business. It's also a relatively new one, and one of the problems is that while many wonderful-sounding claims are made almost every week, there are often caveats and almost nothing has been in use long enough for the long-term effects to be known.

So what follows is a brief – and cautious – guide to some (but by no means all) of the most popular supplements. And to be clear: I don't advise anyone to take anything. That should be your choice and no one else's, a choice that should be informed by your own research and an acceptance that you may be wasting your money as well as possibly risking your health.

In fact, the only safe, proven way to improve your longevity is through diet, exercise and sleep – exactly what I've already outlined in this book.

Having said that, I do take a few supplements myself! If I could take only one, though, it would be hormone replacment therapy or HRT – so I'll start with that.

IT'S YOUR HORMONES...

Dr Erika Schwartz has been one of the most active and influential proponents of HRT for decades. And for decades she was, as she ruefully puts it today, 'screaming in the dark'.

When I first met Dr Schwartz I was in my early 50s and a couple of years into the menopause. Despite being very physically active by then – running, yoga, tennis – and having long stopped smoking, I suffered from drenching night sweats and debilitating daytime hot flushes that were so bad I had to consider carefully each day what to wear to work. For example, anything light coloured was out, because it would inevitably end up with huge sweat marks all over it; but likewise, warm dresses or tops were also out, no matter how cold it might be outside, because once my body started a hot flush, I'd be radiating so much heat you could probably have fried an egg on me.

Even though this was 2016, I didn't discuss it with anyone. That seems extraordinary today, when menopause is such a widely discussed subject, but even as recently as 10 years ago, many women, especially those in the corporate world, just didn't talk about it. They weren't routinely prescribed it either, thanks to something called the Women's Health Initiative. This was what turned out to be a flawed study, published in 2002, that suggested women taking HRT were at increased risk of breast cancer, heart disease, stroke and blood clots. Not surprisingly, it gained huge publicity and scared millions of women – and their doctors – into stopping HRT.

So when I met Dr Schwartz, through a former colleague who'd moved to the US, I was completely taken aback when she asked if I took HRT. 'No, no, I don't need it,' I said breezily. She looked surprised. 'Do you get hot flashes?' she asked. 'Oh yes, very much so,' I said. 'What about night sweats?' 'Drenching ones,' I replied, 'so bad, in fact, that I've taken to covering the bedsheet with towels.'

'Trust me,' she said. 'You need HRT.'

For her to assess me properly meant having a comprehensive blood test to measure not only my hormone levels but various other key biomarkers such as C-reactive protein. I had to have it done privately, which cost an eye-watering £1200. (Why doesn't the NHS offer this to menopausal women? It should, as it flags many potential health dangers, and prevention is so much better than cure.)

But once I started using HRT – estradiol, micronised progesterone, and a small amount of testosterone – my life transformed. The hot flushes disappeared and so did the night sweats. It was like magic. I got my sleep back. I could wear whatever I liked and never had to worry again about turning into a human frying pan.

And now it seems I have even more reason to be grateful to her. Because research by GlycanAge – which you may remember is the company who tested me for my biological age – shows that oestrogen plays a huge role in reducing women's biological age. In one double-blind, placebo-controlled trial published in October 2020,[1] researchers found that when they blocked oestrogen for six months in peri-menopausal women, their biological age *increased by NINE years*. In other words, they aged biologically by almost a decade. When the women were given oestrogen to bring their levels back to where they had been, their biological age went back to where it had been before.

As Dr Schwartz explains over Zoom from her New York office, during our reproductive years we tend to be pretty healthy. And that's mainly because the high levels of sex hormones we produce – oestrogen, progesterone and testosterone – protect us from illness. But once we reach menopause, we are no longer useful in terms of furthering the species. Our hormones disappear. Which results, she says, in one main thing: ageing.

As our levels dwindle, we get some or all of the following: bloating, depression, hot flushes, night sweats, forgetfulness, diminished energy and libido, saggy skin. (And by the way, the same applies to men – see the next section).

'If you don't have hormones,' she explains, 'or if they're out of balance, you get old. You're not going to be able to exercise, you're not going to be able to eat better, you're not going to be able to sleep. You're not going to be able to do anything. That's a way of Mother Nature taking you out.

'I feel hormones are even more important today than 30 years ago, when I first started giving hormone treatment.'

---

1 Effects of estradiol on biological age measured using the glycan age index. *Aging*, 2020 – doi.org/10.18632/aging.104060

I point out that, more than two decades on from what are now accepted as flawed conclusions drawn from the Women's Health Initiative study, some women are still nervous about an increased risk of breast cancer from taking HRT.

Today, the NHS says that the increased risk of breast cancer caused by HRT is 'very low': around five extra cases for every thousand women who take it for five years, and that that risk is usually outweighed by the benefits, which include not just alleviating menopausal symptoms – hot flushes, night sweats, anxiety/low mood, vaginal dryness – but also helping to prevent osteoporosis and maintain muscle strength. HRT also has 'little or no effect' on the risk of coronary heart disease. HRT patches, sprays and gels do not increase the risk of blood clots or stroke. HRT tablets do – but only very slightly.

Dr Schwartz calls the Women's Health Initiative study 'disastrous'.

Out of the thousands of patients she has treated with HRT over the last 30 years, she says, two developed ovarian cancer and one developed breast cancer. She adds that this is a lower number than would be expected for either disease in the population at large, according to statistics.

Nor does she recommend stopping HRT at any point – 'unless you want to get old and sick; if you do want that, then by all means stop.

'But why would you stop taking hormones when you have all the data supporting them? Even the principal investigators of the Women's Health Initiative showed there was NO difference in all-cause mortality between the women on hormones and those on placebo. I personally have been taking HRT now for 28 years. I'm now 74 and have no intention of stopping – none.'

HRT FOR MEN

Yes, men need HRT too. And the only reason this is not better known and more widely discussed, says Dr Schwartz, is that men themselves are too embarrassed to talk about it. They feel that it is shaming – unmanly – to admit that they may need extra testosterone. But the signs are there if you look, she says: the protruding gut and the depression so frequent in middle-aged men are just two of them.

And although her Evolved Science longevity clinics in the US are now treating more and more men, she's noticed that British males are among the most reluctant to concede even the possibility that they may need testosterone. After all, men are proud that they can still father a child in their 80s – although the truth, says Dr Schwartz, is that 80-something men who do so naturally are as rare as women who give birth in their 50s.

Furthermore, it appears that the idea that testosterone supplements increases the risk of prostate cancer is wrong. According to Dr Abraham Morgantaler, an associate clinical professor of urology at Harvard, who has spent decades researching the impact of testosterone in men, there is no evidence that taking it increases the risk.

In fact, the opposite may be true. One of the markers for judging the risk of prostate cancer is PSA – the levels of prostate specific antigen in the blood. Men with normal PSA levels are considered at low risk of prostate cancer. Men with high levels are considered to be at high risk. When Dr Morgentaler started his research, he expected to find that men with normal PSA levels who also had low testosterone might have extra protection against developing the disease. But instead he found that those men went on to develop prostate cancer at the same rate as men whose high levels of PSA put them in the high-risk category.

VITAMINS AND MINERALS

Many experts will tell you that if you're eating a properly balanced diet you will be getting all the vitamins and minerals your body needs.

Try telling that to Bryan Johnson, the 45-year-old multi-millionaire tech tycoon who is currently on a mission to reduce his biological age to 18. And so far he has achieved the fitness of an 18-year-old, the skin of a 28-year-old and the heart of a 37-year-old.

His punishing, expensive regime is so finely calibrated that he is never allowed a cheat day. He goes to bed at 8.30pm every night, eats a carefully curated diet of mostly vegetables, exercises for at least an hour – and takes (by my count, calculated in February 2025 from his daily protocol, which he publishes on his website), at least 45 vitamins, minerals and other supplements every day.

For most of us this is not an option – way too expensive, even if we knew what to take and how much (which Johnson does – everything he takes is calibrated by his medical team exactly to his individual needs).

But while there are many scientists who think vitamins are unnecessary, there are others, top longevity experts among them, who believe that it is extremely difficult to consistently get all the vitamins and minerals your body needs from diet alone. They include David Sinclair, Andrew Huberman and even the self-confessedly cautious Valter Longo, who recommends taking omega-3 and a multivitamin, but only on three days a week.

The decision whether to take vitamins and minerals is one you have to make for yourself.

What I will say is that if you are going to take any supplement, do some careful research first to find out exactly what you're getting, as not all supplements are created equal. Nutrisearch, a company based in Canada, has been evaluating the quality of supplements in America and Canada (not the UK, sadly) for around 20 years, using strict criteria.

Suffice it to say that only a handful of American and Canadian supplement manufacturers achieve a 5-star rating. Those that do are then invited to have every compound in their product independently tested and assessed. The top-performing company listed in the latest edition of their Comparative Guide To Nutritional Supplements is the US company Usana. For that reason I buy most of the supplements I do take – vitamin D, omega-3 and a multivitamin and mineral – from them.

I take vitamin D and omega-3 every day, and a multivitamin and multimineral every other day, at half the dose suggested by Usana. This is because although I believe I am getting the bulk of what I need from my diet, I also know that my diet is not perfect, or at least not every day. Taking them on alternate days at half the dose makes it much more cost effective too.

The other supplements I take are a combined pre- and probiotic, to enhance my gut microbiome; collagen, in the hope that it will help keep some elasticity and firmness in my skin; magnesium and NMN.

Omega-3

A study by the University of Zurich, published in February 2025, found that taking 1g of omega-3 a day slows down biological ageing by up to four months. Omega-3 can also improve heart, brain and eye health, and reduce inflammation.

There have been mixed results from studies looking at whether omega-3 fatty acids improve cardiovascular health. However, a

2021 meta-analysis[2] of 38 trials involving just under 150,000 participants concluded that omega-3 can reduce the risk of heart attacks and strokes, while another, published in the *Alzheimer's & Dementia Journal*,[3] found that 900mg of omega-3 DHA over 24 weeks improved learning and memory in patients with Alzheimer's disease.

Magnesium

Some studies have found that taking a magnesium supplement is good for bone health, and that increasing intake increases bone density in postmenopausal women.[4]

Magnesium also appears to slightly decrease blood pressure, and reduce the risk of heart disease and stroke. There are also claims that it improves sleep, although there is not enough evidence yet to prove that; however, it does improve muscle relaxation.

Turmeric/curcumin

There is no doubt that curcumin, which is found in turmeric, reduces inflammation. That said, there has always been a question mark over its bioavailability – that is, its ability to be absorbed and used by the body. However, a fascinating and rigorous meta-analysis[5] of 66 randomised clinically controlled trials by

---

2 Individual and additive effects of vitamin D, omega-3 and exercise on DNA methylation clocks of biological aging in older adults from the DO-HEALTH trial. *Nature Aging*, 2025 – doi:10.1038/s43587-024-00793-y
3 Beneficial effects of docosahexaenoic acid on cognition in age-related cognitive decline. *Alzheimers Dement.*, 2010 – doi:10.1016/j.jalz.2010.01.013
4 Short-term oral magnesium supplementation suppresses bone turnover in postmenopausal osteoporotic women. *Biol. Trace Elem. Res.* 2010 – doi: 10.1007/s12011-009-8416-8. Epub 2009 Jun 2.
5 Antioxidant and anti-inflammatory effects of curcumin/turmeric supplementation in adults. *Cytokine*, 2023 – doi.org/10.1016/j.cyto.2023.156144

Iran's Shiraz University of Medical Sciences in 2023 found that turmeric/curcumin supplementation positively impacts markers of systematic inflammation and oxidative stress *irrespective of the size of dose or duration of treatment*. This seems extraordinary. The researchers did find 'marginal significant impact association' with increased dosages of curcumin on one marker, TAC (total antioxidant capacity). They also pointed out that their study was in healthy people (as opposed to those suffering from chronic inflammatory conditions, such as osteoarthritis). Despite this, they concluded: 'Overall it could be assumed that turmeric/curcumin improves indices/measurements of inflammation and oxidative stress in individuals with various health status.'

Collagen

Research into collagen's effects on skin appearance is slender at the moment, and what there is tends to be done by companies selling it as a product. But a double-blind placebo-controlled trial conducted by the University of Kiel and the University of San Paolo together with the Collagen Research Institute and Skin Investigation and Technology in Hamburg[6] found that taking just 2.5g a day (considered a low dose – most recommendations are for 10g a day) improved skin elasticity in women of all ages, with significantly greater effects – up to 30 per cent – in women over 50.

If you are going to take it, look for hydrolysed collagen, as this is easier for the body to absorb (you mix it with water and drink it). There is some limited evidence to suggest that marine collagen may be more effective than bovine collagen.

---

6 Oral Supplementation of Specific Collagen Peptides Has Beneficial Effects on Human Skin Physiology. *Skin Pharm. and Phys.*, 2013 – doi. org/10.1159/000351376

Creatine

Bodybuilders have long known that creatine increases muscle and energy. It is also extremely safe to take. But recent claims that it also improves brain function and memory may be overblown. In August 2023, one meta-analysis[7] showed that taking creatine led to 'significant' improvements in memory for people aged 66 and over, while another published in May 2024[8] found no evidence of an improvement in brain cognition. Meanwhile, results from a randomised controlled study published in November 2023[9] showed that it may have a small effect on improving brain function. More research is clearly needed.

NMN – nicotinamide mononucleotide

As I said earlier, the majority of the research into NMN has been in mice. But there are good reasons to believe that similar effects might be found in humans.

The science community is still divided on the benefits of NMN, and until rigorous clinical trials are complete in humans, we can't know for sure who is right. But David Sinclair – who, as I've said before, is one of the world's leading longevity scientists – believes that NMN very likely does have all those same effects, and has been taking it for nine years.

---

7 Effects of creatine supplementation on memory in healthy individuals. *Nutrition Reviews*, 2023 – doi.org/10.1093/nutrit/nuac064
8 Creatine supplementation research fails to support the theoretical basis for an effect on cognition. *Behav. Brain Research*, 2024 – doi.org/10.1016/j. bbr.2024.114982
9 The effects of creatine supplementation on cognitive performance. *BMC Med*., 2023 – https://doi.org/10.1186/s12916-023-03146-5

His father has also been taking it since he was in his 70s and, reports Sinclair, noticed within six months that he was less tired, more alert and outpacing his friends physically.

So what is NMN, exactly? It's a compound found in small quantities in plants, such as broccoli, edamame beans and cucumber, and and has been found to boost production of another compound substance called NAD (nicotinamide adenine dinucleotide).

NAD is involved in many processes in the body, including metabolism, energy production, longevity, DNA repair and immune system function. It's critical to our body – without it we wouldn't make energy and would be dead in less than a minute. But the bad news is that our levels of NAD naturally decrease with age.

Research is still in the early stages, but so far trials in humans suggest that it is safe to take up to 900mg of NMN a day, and that it can increase levels of NAD.

There are ongoing and planned clinical trials aimed at rigorously assessing the efficacy and safety of NMN supplementation across various health outcomes, including its effects on metabolism, cardiovascular health and possibly even cognitive function. A review[10] published in the *International Journal of Molecular Sciences* in September 2024 concluded: 'NMN supplementation acts as a promising approach for improving cardiovascular metabolism health and therapeutic cardiovascular diseases. However, further clinical trials are still needed to explore the mechanism of cardio-vascular protection, appropriate population and optimal dosage for NMN supplementation.'

---

10 Nicotinamide Mononucleotide: Research Process in Cardiovascular Diseases. *Int. J. Mol. Sci.* 2024 – doi.org/10.3390/ijms25179526

The results of a randomised double-blind placebo-controlled clinical trial,[11] published in *GeroScience* in February 2023, were also promising. Of 80 healthy, middle-aged participants (men and women aged 40–65), all those given NMN (three groups of 20, taking it in doses of either 300mg, 600mg or 900mg) showed significant improvements in their levels of NAD, physical endurance (measured with a six-minute walking test), biological age and insulin resistance compared to the 20 who took the placebo. Those on the higher doses of NMN showed greater improvements than those who took only 300mg.

Neither the participants nor the trial staff at the two clinical centres who handed out the capsules (which were identical in every way other than their contents – the placebo contained rice flour) knew whether they were getting the NMN or the placebo. However, it should be noted that of the nine research scientists, three were employed by companies that make NMN (the other six had no conflict of interest).

So it is still very early days and anyone who takes NMN at the moment does so at their own risk. I definitely do *not* make any recommendation for anyone to do so – the safest measure would be to wait at least another 10 years and judge from a great deal more research. Although even then, there would be no means of knowing what long-term side effects there might be.

However, in the interests of full disclosure, I take 1000mg (1g) a day of NMN and have done for the last four years. So far I have suffered no side effects and generally have very high energy. Whether that has anything to do with NMN I cannot be sure,

---

11 The efficacy and safety of β-nicotinamide mononucleotide (NMN) supplementation in healthy middle-aged adults. *Geroscience*, 2023 – doi: 10.1007/s11357-022-00705-1

because I also exercise regularly, eat a (mostly) heathy diet, usually sleep well and drink very little alcohol.

Other longevity supplements:

- **Rapamycin.** This substance mimics the effects of fasting and also inhibits mTor, a set of proteins involved in ageing that regulate growth and metabolisms. But, although it has become a darling of longevity nerds, it is in fact an immune suppressant with unpleasant side effects and getting the dose right is difficult. Bryan Johnson recently stopped taking it, after five years, for this reason.

- **Metformin.** Currently available only on prescription, metformin was developed as a drug to treat type 2 diabetes. Those with type 2 who take it live longer than those with the disease who don't. It also seems to be very safe. Proponents of taking it for longevity, who include David Sinclair, say it appears to decrease the risk of cancer as well as raise NAD levels, inhibit mTor, activate the enzyme AMPK, which restores mitochondria function, improve cardiovascular health and possibly help prevent dementia. However, a critical review published in *Frontiers in Endocrinology* in 2021[12] pointed out that the evidence on the efficacy of metformin as an anti-ageing therapy is mixed and that it is too soon to view it as an anti-ageing treatment. Instead, concluded the authors, people would be better to focus on… diet and exercise!

---

12 A Critical Review of the Evidence That Metformin Is a Putative Anti-Aging Drug That Enhances Healthspan and Extends Lifespan. *Front. Endocrinol.*, 2021 – pmc.ncbi.nlm.nih.gov/articles/PMC8374068/

- **Berberine.** A 2020 meta-analysis[13] found that berberine treatment 'moderately but significantly decreased body weight' by 2kg, as well as BMI and waist circumference, and also reduced levels of C-reactive protein, a key marker of inflammation. David Sinclair says it mimics the effects of metformin.

- **Spermidine.** Much more research is needed but early indications are that spermidine may help promote autophagy and also improve memory.

- **Quercetin.** Many clinical studies have shown that quercetin can be used to treat obesity because of its ability to break down fat cells and improve inflammation. In addition, a 2024 meta-analysis[14] of 20 randomised controlled trials, in which doses of quercetin ranged from 100mg to 3000mg for periods of between two weeks and 12 weeks, found that quercetin supplementation reduced systolic blood pressure (the first number in a blood pressure reading, indicating the pressure in your arteries when the heart beats) and fasting blood glucose (used as an indicator for diabetes or pre-diabetes, this is the level of glucose in your blood when you haven't eaten for at least eight hours), but had no significant impact on cholesterol, triglycerides or diastolic blood pressure.

---

13 The effect of berberine supplementation on obesity parameters, inflammation and liver function enzymes. *Clin. Nutr. Espen*, 2020 – doi: 10.1016/j.clnesp.2020.04.010
14 The effect of quercetin supplementation on the components of metabolic syndrome in adults. *J. of Funct. Foods*, 2024 – doi.org/10.1016/j.jff.2024.106175

- **Fisetin.** Studies in mice have shown that this flavonoid found naturally in strawberries and onions kills senescent cells. This means it could have many benefits in humans; and indeed, in one recent trial[15] in January 2024, it decreased biomarkers in patients with age-related osteoarthritis by an average of 27 per cent. It shows promise, too, for improving inflammation and both cardiovascular and cognitive health, as it crosses the blood-brain barrier. Early studies indicate it is safe to take but much more research is needed.

- **Sodium butyrate** – Butyrate is a short-chain fatty acid produced by the microbes in the gut. If you eat a high-fibre diet, you'll make plenty! It has multiple benefits, from promoting anti-inflammatory processes in the body and brain to improving memory and cognitive impairment, while studies on mice show that it causes significant improvement in learning and memory even in advanced Alzheimer's and after traumatic brain injury and some neurological diseases.[16]

---

15 Fisetin as a senotherapeutic agent: Evidence and perspectives for age-related diseases. *Mech. of Aging and Devel.*, 2024 – doi.org/10.1016/j.mad.2024.111995
16 Butyrate, neuroepigenetics and the gut microbiome: can a high fiber diet improve brain health? *Neurosci. Lett., 2016* – doi: 10.1016/j.neulet.2016.02.009

7
GO FOR IT!

If, like me, you had pre-teen children back in 2012, you might remember a song called 'Dumb Ways To Die'.

It was launched as a rail safety campaign in Australia but thanks to its ridiculously catchy tune and madly eclectic lyrics soon went viral, topping the iTunes charts in 28 countries – displacing Rihanna – and hitting 30 million views on YouTube.

The many foolish methods it outlined of meeting your maker ranged from setting fire to your hair, poking a stick at a grizzly bear, getting your toast out with a fork and doing your own electrical work, interspersed with the refrain:

Dumb ways to die
So many dumb ways to die
Dumb ways to die
So many dumb ways to die

You get the idea. Very silly. And obviously those really are dumb ways to die. But if you think about it, are they any dumber than the way we die in the West, making lifestyle choices that mean we suffer years – even decades – of poor health before gasping our last?

Just how smart is it to live in such a way that you begin to suffer the debilitating effects of diabetes or high blood pressure or heart disease when you reach your early 60s? Because that's when most of us in the UK (61) and US (64) come to the end of our *healthspan* (as opposed to our lifespan).

It means that in England the average man can expect to live out the last 18 years of his life in ill-health before dying at 79, while for the average woman it's even worse – she can expect to die aged 83, after a grim 22 years of deteriorating health.

In the US, where research suggests a staggering four out of five adults over 60 have two or more chronic diseases, men die younger than in the UK, at 74, so can expect 10 years of misery before meeting the Grim Reaper. For women – average age at death, 80 – it's 16.

But it doesn't have to be that way.

When your last surviving parent dies it brings your own life, and death, into sharp focus. That certainly happened to me. Combined with turning 60 – a bleaker, more ominous milestone than I'd anticipated – I felt something close to panic when my father died 18 months later.

I finally understood – viscerally, as opposed to intellectually – that time really was running out; that my life really would end one day, and there was nothing I could do to stop that happening.

But the more I thought about it, the more I realised that there was a better way to look at it. Yes, death comes for us all. But there is so much we can do to make the intervening years, whatever the number, not just less bleak but actively enjoyable.

As I have tried to emphasise throughout this book, it is never too late. Take exercise. Several studies show 12 weeks' strength training is enough to significantly improve muscle in frail, elderly people even in their 90s[1] – and one recent study recorded

---

1 Multicomponent exercises including muscle power training enhance muscle mass, power output, and functional outcomes in institutionalized frail nonagenarians. *AGE*, 2014 –. doi:/10.1007/s11357-013-9586-z

improvements after just eight weeks.

So it really will pay not just to start each of the three-week plans in this book, but to continue with them.

Eighteen months after taking the GlycanAge biological test, I did it again. I can't pretend I wasn't nervous: suppose the first one had been a freak result, or a mix up, or an error by someone in the lab?

By now I was 62. There had been plenty of stress and challenges in my life in the meantime, including, but not limited to, the death of my father.

But again the result came back: 20, emblazoned in a big green roundel, and next to it the words: 'Your biological age is 42 years younger than your chronological age at the time of testing.'

So it seems that what I do really is effective. And this book is my attempt to pass on to you what has worked for me, as I passionately believe every single one of us deserves to be as healthy as possible for as long as possible.

All it takes is a decision to move a little more each day, eat a little less (but more fibre when you do) and rest and sleep more deeply. I hope you'll take not just my word for that, but that of all the distinguished scientists whose work I've explored and drawn inspiration from. These methods work better than any anti-ageing medicine currently available and cost nothing.

Invest in yourself. The benefits of eating more fibre, for example, are so huge that you are actively sabotaging your health if you don't try eating more of it. If the idea of beans and lentils is too off-putting or seems too much like hard work, then start with an apple, a handful of nuts and some avocado on a slice of wholegrain toast and build up from there.

As I was finishing this book I was struck by a remark made by a wonderfully spry and active centenarian in Sydney named Betty

Woodhams, who said her advice to others was never to stop, always look for enjoyment and don't bother with regrets.

'I don't think you can live your life well with regrets,' she said. 'When you make decisions, you make them on what's happening at that time. It's too easy to look back later and say you made a wrong choice. You believed it was the right choice at that time so regretting it won't change it.'

I think she's right. And no matter how out of shape you are, or how old, don't beat yourself up. Resolve instead to treat yourself with kindness. Yes, take responsibility for your actions, but coach yourself as you would your best friend – gently, positively, with a smile and hopefully some laughs. Life's hard enough – why make it harder?

To go back to Deepak Chopra's advice: let go of the drama. Actually, just telling yourself to let go is incredibly helpful. Try it now. Take a deep inhale through your nose, then a long exhale through your mouth. Tell yourself to let go. Do it again, and this time, consciously relax your jaw. Do it again, and consciously relax your shoulders. And again, gently reminding yourself to relax and let go.

You'll realise, when you do, just how tightly you've been holding on – and to what? Not life, or energy, or health. Nothing, in fact, but your own over-thinking mind, which only ever produces more stress, and with it the chronic inflammation that underlies everything from dementia to heart disease.

At an event in 2024 to mark her newly published memoir, Cher told fans that some of her friends complain about turning 40. 'And I say, "Listen, get over yourself. I'd give anything to be 60 again [she was 78 at the time]". You've got to just keep living your life until you die. Keep going for it. You can never give up. Don't let old age get in your way.'

I hope this book will be your guide to shoving old age out of your way for as long as possible.

APPENDIX

EXERCISE PROGRAMME
FOR COMPLETE BEGINNERS[1]
(Devised by Anne Elliott and her team at Middlesex University)

Do this for four weeks to improve your strength, flexibility, balance and endurance before progressing to the three-week plan.

- Do each of these exercises 6 days a week for 4 weeks. It should take you no longer than 15 minutes a day.
- Before you start, stretch your arms in all directions and try to touch all the corners, walls, floor and ceiling in your room. March on the spot, imagine you have a hula hoop around your waist and move your hips. It's important to warm up your muscles before exercise to avoid injury.

---

1 Elliott, M.L., Caspi, A., Houts, R.M., Ambler, A., Broadbent, J.M., Hancox, R.J., Harrington, H., Hogan, S., Keenan, R., Knodt, A. and Leung, J.H., 2021. Disparities in the pace of biological aging among midlife adults of the same chronological age have implications for future frailty risk and policy. *Nature aging*, 1(3), pp.295–308.

Mehmet, H., Yang, A. W., & Robinson, S. R. (2020). What is the optimal chair stand test protocol for older adults? *Disability and rehab.*, 42(20), 2828-2835.

Mroczek, A., Kaczorowska, A., & Kaczmarzyk, M. (2020). Body structure and physical fitness assessed by the Senior Fitness Test: A cross-sectional study in a sample of Polish seniors. *Med. Science Pulse*, 14(4).

Villafaina, S., Polero, P., Collado-Mateo, D., Fuentes-García, J. P., & Gusi, N. (2019). Impact of adding simultaneous cognitive task in the elbow's range of movement during arm curl test inwomen with fibromyalgia. *Clinical Biomechanics*, 65, 110-115.

- Always start within your 'comfort zone' and every time you do the exercise, make it a little bit harder than it was the day before. There are three ways to do this. 1. Add a little more weight. 2. Add a little more time. 3. Add a little more distance.
- Never push yourself to feel pain. You will not improve. In fact, this will set you back because your body then has to fix the damage you have done.
- Intensity. If I asked you how hard an exercise was for you to do from 1 to 10, where 1 was really easy and 10 was the toughest thing ever, you want to be working at a 7 *for you* – not anyone else's 7.

❶ Dancing and walking

Dance to your favourite songs and let yourself really go (no one is watching!) Twirl, jump, bend, wiggle, twist. Start with one song and work towards two songs – around 5 minutes.

Alternate each day with a walk. On your first day, see how far you can get in 5 minutes. On your next walk, see if you can walk a little further in the same time.

❷ Squat

A squat is one of the best ways of strengthening your lower body. There are a number of ways it can be done around the house.

a. Hold onto the front of the sink and without rounding your back lower your bottom as if you are about to sit down. Then pull yourself up. Start with as many as you can do with a rest in between and gradually work up to 8. You may not be able to get down very far to start with so you can work on both the depth of your squat and the number you can do.

b. Put a dining chair against a wall. Stand in front of it so you can feel the front of the chair on the back of your legs. Stretch your arms out in front of you. Move to sit on the chair slowly, keeping your back straight, and stop just as you feel the chair on your thighs. Don't sit down. Hold it for 2 seconds and then stand upright. Repeat. Start with as many as you can do and work up to 10. When this is too easy, try it on your sofa!

❸ Wall sit

Stand against a wall with your feet forward and slide your back down the wall so it looks like you are sitting on an invisible chair. If this is too much, go down as far as you can. You are aiming to hold it for 1 minute, but you will probably have to start with holding it for just 10–20 seconds. This exercise is also very good for reducing high blood pressure if done regularly.

❹ Seated leg raise

This is a great exercise for improving your core strength. Sit back into a dining chair, feet on the floor. Push your belly button back into your spine and lift one leg so that it is parallel to the floor; hold it for a few seconds and feel how it engages your stomach and sides. Then repeat with the other leg. When this feels easy, lift both legs together, but make sure you have engaged your stomach before you make the move. Aim to hold your legs up for 30 seconds.

❺ Boxing

This is one for upper-body strength. Stand in front of a mirror with one foot in front of the other so you feel strong and stable. Hold weights or a couple of 400g tins in each hand. Bend your elbows and bring the weights/tins up towards your face and start punching each arm in turn, aiming at your own face in the mirror. Build up a rhythm and gently twist your body to help you punch a little further out to each side. Try not to let your arms drop. You are aiming to punch continuously for 2 minutes, but initially you may find your arms and shoulders tire after a few seconds. You can increase the amount of time, the number of punches you achieve in a set time or the weights you are holding.

The old adage 'What can be measured can be improved' works well here. It's a good idea to keep a log of what you have achieved each day so you can monitor your own improvement.

INDEX

ACKNOWLEDGEMENTS

I owe an enormous debt of thanks to all the following:

My daughter Isabella, who with typical thoughtfulness, kindness and efficiency found and booked my first 'writing' Airbnb and then spent hours patiently convincing me that the family would not collapse without me while I went away to write this book. My son Luke, whose repeated urging to think harder, go slower and take the time to get it right was invaluable and wise beyond his years. My husband Serge, for enduring, patiently and uncomplainingly, my writing absences, both physical and mental. And to all three for their love and faith.

The many scientists who so generously and good-naturedly gave me their time and whose work really does help make the world a better place. It has been a privilege to meet you and learn from you.

Rebecca Nicolson and Aurea Carpenter, who are not only exceptional, powerhouse publishers but quite simply two of the most talented and nicest people I know.

Rachel, for the lunch that started it all and unstintingly generous advice; Duncan, for inspiring me, motivating me, and making me laugh; and Tony, for continually telling me I could do it.

Ann, for unfailing friendship, support and wise counsel when things got tough.

Jo, Caroline, Aisling, Sally and Susie for their unerring belief and fabulous companionship – which as we now know are not just life-enhancing, but life-extending!

Corinna, who selflessly expanded her laser focus to the science of longevity and sent me a continuous stream of potentially interesting studies and stories; and Sebastian, for his expertise and empathy.

James at 2020 Recordings for making the audio recording not just painless but fun; Katie, Caz, Neale and Colette for rising to the last-minute challenge of getting my photo taken.

Paul Dacre, who among many things taught me you can always do more, and better; my brilliant Editor, Ted Verity, whose incredible capacity for work while remaining unflappable inspired me to keep going; and my wonderful deputy Ciara Dossett, who together with Katharine Spurrier and James Carey kept the show on the road during my various writing 'holidays'. Their good grace and unbeatable (unrepeatable!) humour make work fun – and life, however long, is always better with that.

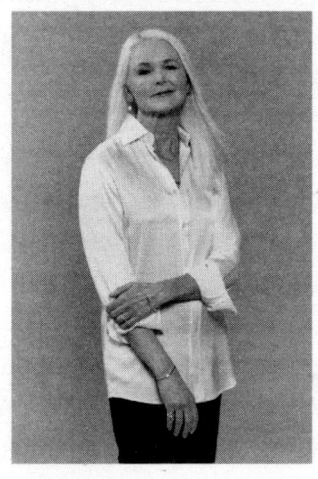

© Neale Haynes

ABOUT THE AUTHOR

Sandra Parsons worked for 13 years at *The Times*, where she launched and edited T2, before becoming a columnist at the *Daily Mail*. She has now been the *Daily Mail*'s literary editor for 15 years. She is also a qualified yoga instructor. She lives in London with her family.